CW00919220

YOU DID

What?

Saying
'No'
To Conventional
Cancer Treatment

YOU DID

What?

———— ∞ ————

Hollie & Patrick Quinn

COBBLESTONE PUBLISHING, LLC

Dedication

With unspeakable gratitude, we dedicate this book...

...to Chanchal and Donnie, master scientists in every sense of the phrase, who prescribed equal doses of wisdom and calm, making Hollie's body *and* spirit well again.

...to "Neighbor Karen," a light in the storm, who perhaps unknowingly recalibrated our compass, and pointed us in the direction of wellness.

...to The Mederi Foundation, whose mission represents the future of healing.

...to all of those who were held back by fear, and suffered unnecessarily, or lost their lives because of it. And to all of those who are presently in the grips of fear, or who might be one day. You have more choices than you know, and you *can* be well again, starting *now*.

Acknowledgments

We wish to thank all the people who helped us make this book a reality. Namely, to our team of editors, who helped us mold the book into its final shape, and to our cover and interior designer, Brion Sausser, who imparted visual beauty to the book and was so very patient with us. And lastly, to all the people who encouraged us over the years to tell our story.

Note to Reader

This book contains information about cancer. The authors are not medical professionals, and neither the authors nor publisher makes warranties, expressed or implied, about the fitness of this information for any particular purpose. Neither the authors nor the publisher advocates any treatment modality. Each reader is strongly urged to consult qualified professional help for medical problems, especially those involving cancer.

Contents

Preface

This book is actually several different stories, all in one. It's part drama, telling the real-life tale of a young woman with a new husband and a newborn child, paralyzed by the fear that cancer had taken life away before she'd had a chance to enjoy it. It's part medical book, organizing and simplifying mountains of complex information needed to make the smartest possible decisions about dealing with cancer. It's part sociology, attempting to explain how mainstream cancer treatment in a modern society like America could have wandered so far from the mission of healing. It's part love story, showing how a young couple simply refused to let a disease separate them, and instead found a way to live long and well together. It's part history, incorporating a bit of the story of how cancer treatment has evolved in America. It's part exposé, revealing what we believe to be an epidemic of medical mistakes being made every day in the treatment of cancer, and also sharing an approach to healing that's better; smarter, healthful, and more scientifically valid.

Perhaps most importantly, it's part inspiration. It's about Hollie Quinn, a 27 year-old woman who, with everything to lose, and in the face of intense fear, complexity, and pressure, rejected conventional treatment for her breast cancer, and lived *well* to tell about it. More than any other goal of ours in writing this book, we want you to know that you can, too, if you're so inclined.

One Voice

We're telling this story together. We've taken quite literally every step of this journey together, from Patrick standing in the PET scan room with Hollie, to sharing in 100% of our lifestyle changes. And the telling of our story in this book is no different. So we'll use "we" or "our" or similar pronouns when we're talking about the journey together, or "Hollie" or "Patrick" (or suitable pronouns) when referring to one or the other of us.

Terminology

This book is about treating cancer. It's about reviewing, analyzing, and choosing between different treatment approaches. We refer to treatments such as surgery, chemotherapy, radiation, and hormone therapy as "Western medicine" or "conventional medicine" or "mainstream medicine." Conversely, we use the term "traditional medicine"[1] broadly to refer to what are commonly called "alternative" or "complementary" medical systems and practices. These ancient healing philosophies include, but are not limited to, herbal medicine, Traditional Chinese Medicine, eclectic medicine, homeopathy, and so forth. Because traditional medicine is inherently holistic in its various forms, and more importantly is tailored to the needs of each person, it often combines more than one healing modality, including elements of Western medicine where appropriate.

Our book cites a fair amount of research in order to share with you the manner in which we came to our decisions. We generally cite research from the past 10-20 years, which is relevant to treatments

---

1. http://en.wikipedia.org/wiki/Traditional_medicine.

currently in use, but we also occasionally cite older studies/research to recount some of the history of cancer treatments.

Chapter-Opening Quotes

Finally, you'll notice that each chapter opens with a quotation. Some of these are taken from well-known people, but many are attributed simply to "Friend." Because Hollie's decision was far from typical, we thought it would be interesting to ask our close friends what they thought about our cancer journey as it was unfolding, and the resulting quotes sit atop most chapter openings.

CHAPTER ONE

Everything To Lose

*"So young and beautiful with many years of living to be done, why, why would a bright young woman with a diagnosis of breast cancer in the 21st century **not** want to take her physicians' advice and go through the treatment that had been recommended?"*

—FRIEND

In August of 2002, the forces of life and death knocked on our door, simultaneously. When we opened the door, there they stood. Our beautiful new daughter, Cassie. And Cancer. Together. Cassie, on the doorstep, in the tight swaddle that she seemed to love being in; and those perfect lips of hers. And cancer—dark, full of fear and despair, beckoning us into its abyss.

Hollie had been diagnosed with Stage 2 breast cancer while 38 weeks pregnant, and just three weeks before her 28th birthday. It was an entirely surreal time, with all the intensely joyful anticipation of a madly-in-love couple's first child, violently colliding with the hammer-in-the-face news that Hollie had cancer, and a pretty serious case, at that. It was like one of those renditions of a bad dream that you see in the movies, where someone's walking along amidst beautiful scenery, and then the blue sky and flowers and other signs of tranquility are slowly replaced with weeds, and darkness, and ominous music. And so much fear. They really should re-classify cancer as a type of paralysis, for all the emotional rigor mortis that it causes when you find out you have it.

We had been planning a natural birth, attended by a midwife in partnership with Hollie's OB-GYN. But those plans were smashed by the diagnosis. To us, cancer was like one of those cyborgs from futuristic sci-fi movies—cold, mechanical, artificial; clinical, intellectual, cynical. Nothing seemed natural to us any more, including the tumors in Hollie's breast, or the bits of cancer seeping into her lymphatic system in her armpit. The doctors induced Hollie's labor at 6pm the same day that the diagnosis had been confirmed. After an emotionally and physically exhausting night, Cassie was born just before 10am the next day. Then they packed Hollie's breasts in ice, and forbade breast feeding. It was supposed to make the upcoming surgery easier, and the doctors were of course expecting that Hollie would be following a conventional treatment protocol, which would not allow for breast feeding. It was just one of the many ways in which Mother Nature was asked to leave the room.

We were literally being ripped in half, emotionally, constantly getting pulled back and forth between hazy happiness about the dawning of our lives, and the thick darkness of fear that it would all end in Hollie's untimely death from cancer. And though we found moments to laugh, and smile, and kiss, and cuddle, we most vividly remember the fear. There was fear all around us, not the least of which was on the faces, and in the words, of the people in white coats who were caring for us. The rush to surgery, the breasts-on-ice, the reminders that cancer in young people is always more aggressive, the imploring to start chemotherapy and radiation as soon as possible.

Everywhere, fear. Eventually, all that fear elicited a powerful force within us, one that drove us in the direction of healing, and hope, just as powerfully as fear pulls you into despair when you have cancer.

We would later learn that, as dark as were these first weeks after the diagnosis, they wouldn't be the worst part about having cancer. As we wandered through the experience, dazed but determined, and always with this powerful intuition that there was a better way, we would soon find ourselves at a fork in the road, a moment of choice that most people with cancer never find. One path led to conventional cancer treatments—chemotherapy, radiation, hormone therapy. There was a good deal of hope on that path, but, also, sickness. Illness and broken bodies when things went "well," and utterly miserable death when they didn't.

The other path led to a smarter, safer way to deal with cancer. But at first this path was almost impossible for us to make out. Hollie, like most cancer patients, had an oppressive sense that she simply had no choice but to listen to the advice of her doctors, that there was only one path back to the normalcy she so desperately craved to feel once again. And all of these feelings were intensified by the fact that we were utter rookies when it came to understanding wellness, let alone traditional medicine. As we agonized about which treatment decision to make, it took us months to be able to see this better path clearly. All the while, though, we could see the horizon to which it led, and it was beautiful. It was a thoroughly, deeply healthy life, *including* the treatment. And that gave us the most uplifting hope we'd ever experienced, and helped us persevere, so that we could cut away the thicket of confusion surrounding that path, to see a clear and safe way back to health.

As we stood at that crossroads, we had everything to lose in making the wrong choice. The wrong choice would leave a devastated, widower husband, and a motherless child. One of our dear friends summed up rather neatly the conundrum we faced as we thought about going down that other path. "Why would a bright young woman with a diagnosis of breast cancer in the 21st century *not* want to take her physicians' advice and go through the treatment that had been recommended?"

Everything to lose, indeed. And yet we did end up going down that other path, and we lived *well* to tell about it.

CHAPTER TWO

The Cancer Canary

"*Orthodox medicine rarely focuses on the immune system as a means of preventing or curing cancer. In fact, orthodox medicine urges women to detect and treat cancer with techniques known to suppress the immune system.*"

– SUSUN S. WEED, AUTHOR

Too many people have cancer today. The canary in the cancer coal mine died a long time ago, but we mostly failed to notice. In the 21st century, we tend to suffer from "paralysis of the analysis," whereby we can't see the forest of truth because we're standing too close to the statistical trees in front of us. As an economist once said, "Numbers lie, trust the eye." The incidence of breast cancer has increased virtually non-stop since the middle of the 20th century, from a rate of 1 in 20 fifty years ago[1], to 1 in 8 today. Overall, 1 in 2 men, and 1 in 3 women, will be diagnosed with some form of cancer in their lifetimes. At current trends, these rates are expected to *double* in the coming decades.[2] And the modern lifestyle causes it. When people from non-Western cultures come to live in places like the U.S., within a generation they face the same risk of developing cancer as

---

1. S. J. Cutler, Barbara Christine, T. H. C. Barclay, "Increasing incidence and decreasing mortality rates for breast cancer," *Cancer*, 28, no. 6 (1971): 1376-180.

2. http://www.medscape.com/viewarticle/551998.

their native-born neighbors, even though the cancer risks in their homelands were much, much lower.

And the worst part is, that's *not* the bad news. The worst part about cancer is what happens *after* your diagnosis. Namely, the "treatment." It doesn't have to be that way, although it's understandable that we think it does. When you've got highly educated doctors telling you it has to be that way, telling you that this treatment or that treatment is the only choice for you, then that's going to sound pretty convincing. Especially when you're *scared to death*. But, it turns out you *do* have choices. There's a pretty good chance your doctor is dead wrong about the cancer treatment he or she is recommending to you or a loved one. Our doctors in Los Angeles were all fiercely intelligent people. And they were completely wrong about what our options were when we found out Hollie had cancer. It turns out you may *not* need to follow your doctor's treatment advice. In fact, it turns out that doing so could be a really, really bad decision on your part. We were just lucky enough, and just brave enough, to disagree with our doctors. And the result was like winning the lottery. We embarked on an incredible journey of healing and happiness.

Cancer Treatment Today

The American Cancer Society estimated that in 2009, there would be approximately 1,479,350 new cases of cancer, and more than 562,000 deaths from cancer, which is more than 1,500 deaths each day. In the United States, cancer accounts for nearly one out of every four deaths.[3]

---

3.   http://www.cancer.org/downloads/STT/500809web.pdf.

There's a suffocating amount of dishonesty on the part of the cancer treatment industry. We hold all medical care providers— traditional/alternative, or conventional—to the same high standards. Truth and the hippocratic oath should be guiding principles for doctors, but they rarely are. The sad reality is that, in the area of cancer treatment, it's actually very difficult to find a thinking doctor. The herd mentality is completely unexpected, but it's there.[4]

After our initial consultations with more than a dozen medical practitioners, we assembled a team that has always included a couple of conventional medical doctors—one oncologist, and one surgeon (the one who performed Hollie's lumpectomy). Despite some of the admittedly harsh words we sometimes have for doctors, the reality is that there's a very strong pragmatic theme in our story. It's a simple case of using the right tool for the job. Beyond the skills of surgical precision (arguably Western medicine's greatest talent) and diagnostic technology (arguably its second greatest talent), the tools that conventional docs wield are just not very effective. So, we use medical doctors for what they're good at, and traditional healers for the rest. Again, this is a growing trend, and in the coming years it will be commonplace, especially for serious illnesses like cancer. Today's mainstream treatments for cancer will be looked upon as barbaric and unsophisticated. After our experience with cancer, we couldn't agree more with the words of Dr. Andy Weil: "I do think that one day, we will look back on the chemotherapy era and look at

4. Here we're referring specifically to the "standard of care," which is a troubling form of groupthink in conventional medicine, and which we discuss more in later chapters.

it the same way we looked on the way we used to treat mental illness 100 years ago."[5]

Every year in America, tens of thousands of women are given treatments for breast cancer that are either unnecessary, or ineffective, or both.[6] These are medical mistakes. Most women will merely be made violently ill by these mistakes. But treatment mistakes also may cause severe and often permanent damage to their bodies, when they would have returned to health following breast cancer even without the harmful treatments. Some will die as a result of these mistakes, when they might otherwise have lived.

When Hollie was diagnosed with breast cancer, all of our conventional physicians said exactly the same thing: "Hollie, you *need* chemotherapy, radiation, and hormone treatment." It wasn't optional or preventive, they all concurred. One doctor also said she needed extensive additional surgery, beyond the lump removal she had immediately after diagnosis. And this particular doctor went so far as to say, coldly, (and we're quoting here), "you'll probably die if you don't."

And they were all wrong. *All of them.* And they're all immensely smart people, practicing cancer treatment at premiere, major metropolitan locations like UCLA Medical Center and Cedars Sinai Medical Center. And yet they were wrong about Hollie, and they may be wrong about you, too, if you have cancer. That's why we want you to read this book. We want you to *choose* your treatment, **consciously,**

---

5. *Larry King Live*, 10/25/05, http://transcripts.cnn.com/TRANSCRIPTS/0510/25/lkl.01.html.

6. The same problem applies to other cancers as well, but the problem is most pronounced with breast cancer.

whether the treatment is recommended by a conventional doctor, naturopathic doctor, herbalist, or any other health practitioner.

There's no denying that there is very good justification for utilizing certain conventional treatments in certain specific situations. For example, the herbal medicine clinic that treated Hollie will frequently use very finely tuned chemotherapy formulations under certain circumstances. Again, these decisions boil down to using the right tool for the job.

Let us formally state for the record that we are not against all conventional treatment all of the time. In all honesty, such an absolutist attitude would be foolish, and life-threatening. But by and large, the conventional cancer treatment industry uses a one-size-fits-all, assembly-line approach to treating cancer patients. The philosophy and practices of the conventional cancer treatment industry are best summarized by Dr. Susan Love: "Unfortunately we are left guessing on the basis of probabilities that are not individualized. This usually means that we overtreat, fearing that we might miss someone who could benefit."[7]

Tipping Point

There's an increasingly loud chorus of voices pointing out the flaws of today's cancer treatment industry. And it is an industry, complete with standardized, boilerplate "treatments," professional associations, and lots and lots of money powering it all. What's interesting is that, more and more, there are voices from *within*

---

7. Susan M. Love, M.D., *Dr. Susan Love's Breast Book, Third Edition, Fully Revised* (Cambridge: Perseus Publishing, 2000), 388.

the cancer treatment industry questioning the entire system. In fact, in one survey, 75 percent of oncologists said that if they had cancer, they would not participate in chemotherapy trials due to its "ineffectiveness and its unacceptable toxicity."[8] Read that again: *Seventy-five percent.*

Dr. Kenneth Forror was a surgeon who routinely recommended chemotherapy to patients. But "with colon cancer at age sixty, [he] was told by his oncologist he would only live one more year, provided he started with chemotherapy or radiation immediately. He refused treatment. He is now retired at age eighty-three."[9] Dr. Lorraine Day had an advanced, aggressive form of breast cancer, but her medical training, and intuition, told her that she would certainly die if she succumbed to conventional treatments, which she resolutely refused, and eventually cured herself of cancer naturally.[10]

Despite the slowly changing attitudes about cancer treatment, make no mistake about it—the cancer business is still a juggernaut. It has tremendous force and speed. But it can, and should, be derailed. It's going in the wrong direction, and fast. In order to change the direction of a moving force like that, it would require an equally powerful force. That force is the power of choice. It's no coincidence that one of the first things you hear after being diagnosed with cancer is, in so many words, that you have no choice but to follow the advice of your doctors. That's not at all correct, and doing so can kill you.

---

8. John Robbins, *Reclaiming Our Health* (Tiburon: HJ Kramer, 1998), 240.

9. "Surgeon Refuses Chemotherapy," *Well Being Journal, Special Edition: Healing Cancer Naturally* (2000): cover page.

10. Lorraine Day, M.D., "Cancer Doesn't Scare Me Anymore," video, http://www.drday.com/.

Doctors will usually say that you have no choice, and that you must follow their recommendations. We aren't saying that you must follow our way either. Instead, the message we want to convey is that you have treatment choices and we want to encourage you to be your own personal advocate. Look at *all* the different treatment options (not just the ones offered by your medical doctors under the standard of care), their actual success rates, and the ways in which the treatments affect your body. For instance, does the treatment kill the cancer? Does it use one pathway to destroy the cancer, or does it target multiple pathways? Does it do any other damage to the body? Does it improve the functioning of the immune system? Then ask yourself, which approach makes the most sense to you? At the end of the day, you must choose the route that is best for *you*, not the route that someone is ordering you to take, especially when threatening you with death as your only other alternative. And as we said earlier, above all else we encourage you to hold your healers, whatever their background, to the same high standard—you deserve *clear, convincing evidence* that your treatments are safe and effective *for you as an individual.*

CHAPTER THREE

Discovery

"Of all the illnesses, diseases, and disasters in the world, I think I am most afraid of cancer because of the helplessness associated with it."

—FRIEND

Hollie met her cancer on the evening of Sunday, August 4, 2002. This was the beginning of that schizophrenic period where life and death were with us every day. But life alone was in the air that evening. The anticipation of life, really. Our daughter Cassie was due to be born in about 2 weeks. We'd just returned from our last birthing class, where we'd been eager students of an expert in ushering in life—a midwife of some 40 years' experience. During the class, she had been, unknowingly, training us for our cancer journey. She taught us calm in the face of another potentially difficult, even possibly life-threatening, experience—childbirth. She showed how the many seemingly frightening things that occur during childbirth are a normal and natural part of the process, to be welcomed as milestones on the way to victory for Mother Nature. Looking back, we recalled how she would talk about routinely delivering babies at 42 and 44 weeks, without any of today's worries that the baby would be "too big," or the mother would experience "failure to progress."

Unbeknownst to her, she was the first of many would-be cancer coaches in our lives, all of whom taught us to be calm in the face of cancer, and to realize that cancer, like the almost indescribable tribulation of delivering a child, is a part of us, to be embraced, and not something to be obscured with fear-based over-treatment.

Hollie was getting ready for bed that night, when her hand brushed across her right breast, and she felt, for the first time, a hard lump. It introduced itself as cancer immediately. Like a lawyer in a tense courtroom moment, Hollie had a quick sidebar conversation in her head, telling herself it was nothing. But the judge glared down at her, and she knew then, in the pit of her stomach, that it was something. She called to Patrick to come investigate. Ever the calm one, he assured her it was nothing, though it was certainly hard and "sticky." Unlike a cyst that melds and collapses, this mass was obstinate, refusing to give way to Patrick's nudging it around, which we later learned was the textbook definition of a malignant tumor. Still, with virtually all of medical knowledge just a Google visit away, Patrick did some quick searching, and assured Hollie that it was probably just a clogged milk duct, or at worst a benign fibroadenoma, and then encouraged her to rest up for the festivities of the coming weeks, which might begin at any moment. But while Hollie wanted to believe Patrick, she remained fearful and had a deep, sickening feeling that she knew the truth. We agreed to call the midwife and OB-GYN in the morning, just to be sure.

Being 38 weeks pregnant, it was common for Hollie to get up a lot during the night. And each time she did that night, she'd reach down to check, in hopes it would be gone. But of course it was there to stay, at least for a time.

The next morning, after Patrick left for work, Hollie called our midwife, who agreed over the phone that it was probably just some pregnancy-related cyst, or perhaps an unhappy milk duct. But she invited Hollie to her office anyway (where she shared space with our OB-GYN), to take a quick, closer look, just to be sure. After just a few seconds of examining the tumor, the midwife called in the OB-GYN, who quickly moved Hollie to a room with an ultrasound machine, and then called in his associate to get a second set of eyes on the white blob with seeming tentacles, and calcifications[11], on the screen. With each passing moment, and all within about 15 minutes of Hollie's arrival at the office, the tone was getting more and more serious. The facial expressions had already said what the biopsy report would later state. And then, within minutes of first encountering Hollie's cancer, the OB-GYN and his associate performed a needle biopsy.

So here you are. You have cancer. An unwelcome guest, for sure. And then someone comes along and stabs the guest, repeatedly, and then tells you to go home and sit with it for a few days, while you wait for test results. Cancer *can* go away peacefully, if you know how to ask it to do so. But we start the relationship off badly right from the start. At the time, however, we weren't aware of any of this. So, we went home with our guest, whom we'd just knifed, and sat with it for a few days while we waited for the phone to ring. Talk about awkward.

Mind you, we didn't have this benign, we-met-a-new-friend-

---

11. Calcifications are small bits of calcium that can appear within the soft tissue of the breast. Calcifications are not breast cancer, but sometimes they are an indication of a precancerous condition. http://breastcancer.about.com/od/mammograms/p/calcifications.htm.

today attitude about Hollie's cancer at first. We began this journey innocent and completely uninformed. Our knowledge of cancer was elementary. Our awareness of traditional medicine was practically non-existent. As we said in chapter 1, we initially viewed Hollie's diagnosis in the same way most others did—as nothing less than a visit from the grim reaper. But this was one of the most important lessons we learned along the way. The notion of cancer as some foreign invader forms the very foundation of our problems in dealing with it. It gives rise to the practice of waging "war" against it, and justifies the use of the weapons of mass destruction that are conventional treatments. And worst of all, it blinds us to the fact that it's a part of us, a product of our bodies and our biologies and our environments. A natural process, even. Thus, rather than addressing the underlying imbalances that cause our cancers, with the body and its amazing immune system as the most powerful tools at our disposal, we instead sacrifice our bodies as collateral damage in a cancer jihad. And newly diagnosed patients are especially vulnerable to taking on this mindset. The "let's go to war" mentality is a misguided but understandable emotional surrogate that fills the void in your confidence, and basic sense of well-being, created by a cancer diagnosis. But we've been engaged in this struggle with cancer for a half-century, and it's time to stop. It's time to make peace with cancer.

We took that first step towards making peace with Hollie's cancer when it greeted her for the first time on that Sunday evening in 2002.

CHAPTER FOUR

Diagnosis

"You had just given birth to a beautiful baby girl and I was so afraid you would not be able to see her grow up."

—FRIEND

For the 48 hours following the needle biopsy, we floated in a kind of limbo between two lives, one before cancer, and the other a lifelong healing path. We returned to our routine tasks, with Patrick back at work as a software programmer, wrapping up projects in preparation for time off for the baby's arrival, and Hollie continuing to prepare for the big day. We mostly ignored the possibility that the pathology report would reveal the tumor to be malignant. Sure, we had a couple of "What if?" conversations during our nightly long walks, but we dismissed the possibility as quickly as it came up. No way. We weren't even thirty yet. Hollie was *twenty seven*, and our first child was on the way. Doesn't happen. *Can't* happen, can it?

And all the while, that cancer sat quietly in Hollie's breast, irritated from the piercings of the biopsy needle, but, still willing to cooperate. Only later would we learn just how important it is to work *with* your cancer, and never against it.

Wednesday, August 7, 2002

Patrick went to work as usual in the morning, and, having just gone on maternity leave from her job, Hollie did some things around the house, then laid down on the couch for a little rest just before noon. Hollie heard the phone ring. In one of her first and clearest moments of intuition, a skill that would later become an important tool in getting well again, she remembers thinking, "I'm not going to answer that, because this is going to be my last chance to rest for a while." She laid there for another five minutes or so and then went upstairs to listen to the message waiting on the answering machine. It was her OB/GYN, asking her to call him back. He said, "Tell the nurse to interrupt me if I'm with another patient." Even in her stupor of denial, Hollie knew that wasn't a good sign.

She slowly dialed her doctor's number, and he got on the phone and began right away with, "I got the test results back...and it's a malignancy." He proceeded to talk about inducing labor, and how he was going to try to give Hollie as natural a birth as possible, as this had always been her wish. Hollie heard words and phrases like "lymph nodes," "must perform more tests," and "treatments," but it all blurred together. The doctor asked Hollie to come to the office as soon as she was ready.

A few miles away, in a cubicle in downtown Los Angeles, an emotional earthquake was about to shake Patrick's world. The phone on his desk rang, pulling him away from his computer monitor, and the logical, predictable programming code that was laid out on it. It was the last bit of certainty he would see for some time.

"Hello, this is Patrick."

Silence. And then a quivering, halting breathing sound, as Hollie tried to catch enough breath to be able to say the words. But she couldn't actually say them. The fear had literally taken her breath away, leaving her only with the ability to shriek violently.

"IT'S CANCER!!" she screamed into the phone. Patrick's personal 10.0-magnitude shaker had just struck.

"What?!" he said firmly. "Who did you talk to?"

"THE DOCTOR!" She spoke as if she had a knife in her abdomen. And then she lost the capacity even for that arrested speech, and just sobbed uncontrollably on the phone. Certain events in Patrick's life had prepared him for a moment like this, and he drew upon every morsel of that strength now.

"Honey, it's going to be OK. I want you to focus on just one thing, and that's breathing. You've got to try to calm yourself down for the baby. I'll take a cab home right away. Remember to breathe, sweetheart—in through your nose, out through your mouth. I love you."

She never really spoke again on the call. Patrick's words, though, were just enough to connect her to the budding life in her belly, and to restore the slightest sense of being OK. She tried to breathe. In a moment of protest against the chaos that had just unfolded, Patrick set the phone down gently in its cradle, and sat and stared for a brief moment. "Where does this road take us?" he thought to himself.

The fact that his co-workers were aware Hollie was pregnant was the perfect cover to allow him to exit quickly, and without anyone knowing what that phone call was about.

"Hey, I've got to run. Something may be happening with Hollie," he called out as he moved through the cubicles towards the elevator, doing his best to paint a smile on his face. His coworkers smiled with anticipation as they looked up from their desks. Standing on the street waiting for a cab, his mind worked to process the thoughts racing through it. A varsity athlete through high school and college, almost-a-clinical-psychologist by training, and a programmer by trade. *Perfect.* On the 45-minute ride home, he psyched himself up for the "big game" ahead, began preparing strategies to deal with Hollie's mental and emotional state, and methodically ran through checklists in his mind of next steps, possibilities, and so forth.

Hollie slipped into numb pragmatism. The daughter of a Harvard-educated Chief Financial Officer, and a public policy analyst by training and by trade. *Perfect.* "Well, I'm going to have a baby today," she thought to herself, "so I should take a shower." She couldn't feel the water. The fear was like anesthesia.

When Patrick opened the door at home, the house was quiet. He sprinted upstairs, moving in the direction of the crying. He found Hollie *in the closet*, curled up on the floor. Cancer was winning this round. She was down for the count, already emotionally, mentally, and physically spent. As Patrick stood over her, the underdog spirit took over. "This is the last time we're going down," he thought to himself.

But for that moment, he got down on the floor with her, and cried. This was actually the beginning of treatment, expelling all that fear and heavy emotion, in order to allow better feelings to take their place. They soon would, and feelings more exhilarating than we possibly could have imagined at that point in time. But it would take us a while to get there.

We cried and hugged for what seemed like an hour, but what was actually about 15 solid minutes, on the floor of that closet. "This is the smallest room in our house," joked Patrick. "We should probably get out of here now." We were together again, and the energy from that fusion of our spirits lifted us off the floor, and would continue to support us through everything that was coming. Every conversation discussing options. Every doctor's office. Every test. Every fear.

Patrick first broke the news to Hollie's best friend since childhood, and also called another very close friend to help spread the word. He called her parents, too, who lived nearby. They arrived with lunch in hand, and we began discussing the next steps. We tried our best to keep the conversation light, but the presence of cancer filled the room. "How's your turkey? Can you pass the tumor? SORRY!—I meant salt!"

After lunch, we drove to the OB/GYN's office. Our midwife met us at the door and enveloped Hollie in a big hug. Deep sadness filled the office as the entire staff looked on with sympathetic, mostly moist eyes. The clearest sign that we worship blindly at cancer's altar of fear is the reaction of those around you when you have it. The mood in that office was *exactly* the same as if someone had already actually died. It was a vibe of inevitability. Sure, there was tremendous empathy on the part of the most excellent staff in that office, and we'll always be deeply appreciative of those hugs and tears that day. But this was one of the first signs of how clearly we need to stop kneeling in fear to cancer. There was quite literally life inside Hollie that day, as there is inside every person with cancer. But life was asked to leave the room, at least temporarily. Fear prevailed, and fear is anti-healing. And thus it's in these very first moments of having cancer that we turn away from healing, and most of us never turn back from these missteps in the direction of disease.

In the coming days, we were swept up by the conventional medicine juggernaut. Everything was a rush. There was virtually no deliberation. No calm calculation. The recommendation was to induce immediately, and then move right away to testing and surgery to remove the tumor and begin to explore its spread, if any. We made serious decisions with breathtaking speed, all powered by fear, even before we knew anything about the nature of Hollie's cancer. A baby's gestation was interrupted, breastfeeding her forbidden, Hollie's breasts packed in ice to stop the unnatural engorgement that would result from not feeding her child—yet more evidence of how cancer holds sway over the minds of even experienced physicians. But we weren't yet ready to be in charge of our health, and so we went along willingly with it all.

We left the doctor's office and headed straight to Cedars Sinai Medical Center. The staff there had gotten cancer's memo, so to speak, and recreated the ominous mood of the OB/GYN's office. Induction began at 6pm. By 10pm, Hollie was barely 1 cm dilated, and the doctor then broke her water bag with a tool that looked identical to a knitting needle. Without the natural cushion of the water bag, Cassie's tiny but bone-hard skull sunk deeply into Hollie's cervix, setting off very painful, intense, rapid contractions. It was an early lesson of the costs of being out of step with Mother Nature, and one that Hollie wouldn't soon forget.

We spent the next eight hours trying to remain focused on the training from our childbirth classes—breathing and meditation, massage, changing positions often, walking the halls frequently. We found a surprising number of moments of calm throughout the night, even levity. Hollie did an incredible job of focusing on the task at hand, when everyone, including herself, knew very well that her mind was constantly being pulled towards fear. It was the longest night of her life.

Thursday, August 8, 2002

By 6am the next day, the unnatural labor hadn't accomplished much, other than to exhaust Hollie in every way—physically, mentally, emotionally. She was 2 cm dilated, numb, and deeply depressed from her diagnosis the day before. Patrick huddled with the midwife, knowing he had to get some rest for his bride soon. They decided to order an epidural, followed by a Pitocin injection, to move the labor along. Hollie gave all the input of a comatose person at that point. It was as if Patrick were issuing orders via medical power of attorney.

The contractions picked up quickly and strongly, which we could tell only from watching a computer monitor, since the epidural had mostly paralyzed Hollie from the mid-section down. It was an example of conventional medicine's masking powers, at their very best. Something as intense as delivering a child, and Hollie was barely present.

Over the next three hours, classical music played quietly in the room. The midwife waited attentively and serenely in a chair. Patrick fell asleep in another chair next to Hollie's bed. Hollie laid on her side and began crying gently. At one point, a nurse from a new shift came in, apparently without an update from the previous shift, and said, "Oh, honey, don't cry. Women have babies all the time." Nobody said a word. The midwife got up and handed Hollie a tissue.

By about 9am, Hollie had dilated to 10 cm, and since the single-injection epidural (versus a drip) had begun to wear off, Hollie was beginning to feel the natural urges of labor again, and wanted to push. About 45 minutes later, at 9:46am, Cassie Chapin Quinn was born. She was our angel of wellness, having helped usher Hollie's cancer to a quick manifestation and discovery. Hollie turned to Patrick and said, "Yesterday was the worst day of my life, and today is the best." We hadn't yet turned away from cancer, but this was the first time Hollie at least looked over her shoulder in the direction of life. It was a start.

After several hours in the delivery room with our new bundle, another important moment in our journey. The hospital happened to have a lot of maternity patients that day; so many, in fact, that they had to move new mothers to other floors. It just so happened that Hollie was transferred to the oncology ward. The air was thick with death and dying, and the hallways were crowded with people suffering from cancer, every one of them bald and gaunt. Hollie remembers thinking to herself that she would soon be one of them. Little did we know that, deep down, this was one of her first moments of resolution to choose a different path. We held new life in our arms, and yet were surrounded with death. The contrast couldn't have been more stark. The choices before us were starting to crystalize already.

Our ride on the bullet train of "modern" medicine continued apace, with blood tests, scans, meetings with surgeons, medical oncologists, radiation oncologists, genetic counselors, and so forth. We mostly left Cassie behind with family and friends during all of this activity, which saddened Hollie. Some time later, in a meeting with one of our traditional practitioners, during which we were reviewing our early treatment (before we'd begun working with the traditional folks), he mentioned effortlessly that he would have preferred to have Hollie be with her baby, breastfeed, and recover from delivery before beginning any (even natural) treatment. It was the starkest possible contrast to our experience with conventional medicine. In looking back, we were instinctively clinging to life in wanting to be with Cassie more. An angel indeed, and with impeccable timing.

Less than two weeks later, Hollie had a lumpectomy, along with a sentinel node biopsy in order to start to gauge the spread of the cancer through her lymphatic system. It was the last conventional medicine that we accepted, and, despite the relative success of surgery in "curing" cancer, even this intervention is one that Hollie now says she wouldn't do if she had a chance to do it all over again.

Hollie's recovery from the surgery was somewhat difficult (especially considering she had a newborn to care for), starting with some vomiting from the anesthesia following surgery, and continuing with more than a year of nerve pain down her right arm. It was, however, the easiest part of what we would be facing in the next six weeks.

CHAPTER FIVE

Is This As Good As It Gets?

"I know many people that have been diagnosed with cancer and gone through many years of radiation and/or chemo and suffering trying to get better only to find out that it was never gone and kept coming back stronger and stronger. That is why I was devastated and so scared when I found out you had it. I pictured you suffering trying to fight it through the poisoning of chemo and radiation. I honestly hadn't heard of anyone trying to fight it any other way."

—FRIEND

"**P**rimum non nocere." It's a Latin phrase, meaning "First, do no harm," and it's part of the Hippocratic Oath that medical doctors *used to* take routinely. In recent decades, various modern versions began replacing the classic versions (or the oath was just discarded entirely as part of medical school training), and nearly all of the new ones are scrubbed of references to this promise to avoid causing harm.[12] Indeed, some suggest that, for cancer in particular, the new mantra for doctors is "primum succurrere"—"First, hasten to help."[13] A fearful rush to do *something*, anything, is the hallmark of modern cancer treatment.

---

12. http://en.wikipedia.org/wiki/Hippocratic_Oath.
13. http://en.wikipedia.org/wiki/Primum_non_nocere.

Well, haste makes waste, as they say, and the cancer industry in America is a vast wasteland of toxic and largely ineffective treatments. *Everywhere*, there is harm. As our conventional doctors presented treatment options to us in 2002, what stood out the most was how harmful all of the treatments were, and especially chemotherapy. One of the first books we purchased was the popular *Breast Book* by Dr. Susan Love, and it's none other than Dr. Love who referred derisively to the "big 3" conventional cancer treatments (surgery, radiation, chemotherapy) as "slash, burn, poison." All of these are run-of-the-mill medical treatments, in that they only mask the symptoms of cancer, and do literally *nothing* to address the underlying causes of cancer. "Remember that radiation and chemotherapy are themselves mutagenic and carcinogenic."[14]

We had one big advantage in dealing with the fear and confusion we faced—we were both trained social scientists, having met in graduate school at the University of Chicago. Digging through mountains of even very complex information was neither new nor daunting to us. In fact, it provided a welcomed distraction. In the weeks after Hollie's surgery, we shifted into an intense research mode. We purchased dozens upon dozens of books, and obtained copies of medical journals and articles from the conventional oncologists with whom we were meeting. We tracked down a great many citations as well, wanting to get to the original source of information and data whenever we could. And we did this on a full-time basis, with Patrick taking a leave of absence from work, and Hollie already on maternity

---

14. Andrew Weil, M.D., *Spontaneous Healing* (New York: Ballantine Books, 1995), 336.

leave. For two solid months, we compiled information, questioned it relentlessly, and worked to fill in gaps in the information we were gathering wherever we found them.

The biggest problem you face when you have cancer isn't the particular form of cancer you have. It's trying to make sense of what you're being told about cancer—about your chances for survival, about treatment options, and so forth. There's an illusion, when you're sitting in your doctor's office getting advice, that it's the best possible and most honest advice. It's not. And we admit that it's *very* hard to come to grips with the fact that something as important as society's cancer treatment system could be so flawed. But it is. And you *must* know this if you should have cancer. We learned it the hard way, at the same time we were dealing with the devastation of Hollie's diagnosis, and so the lessons are deeply ingrained in us. And we feel that we have to share the naked truths we saw after stripping away misinformation and fear, in the hope that we can all start making much better choices in the face of cancer.

When you look closely and clearly at the data, there simply isn't good evidence to support doing conventional treatments, especially given how much damage they cause to the body. What we were finding is that, in particular for breast cancer, the treatments were more dangerous than the disease itself. We were learning that the vast majority of women either don't need the treatments they get, or, the treatments only end up making their cancers worse, all the while destroying the body's primary tool for healing cancer—the immune system.

Despite what we were seeing about the double-whammy of

ineffectiveness and harmfulness on the part of conventional cancer treatment, we hadn't yet answered the question that probably haunts everyone with doubts about conventional treatments—"If not that, then what?"

In the course of our research, we were uncovering a wealth of information about "complementary" and "alternative" approaches to cancer. But this represented our very first exposure to these views of how to deal effectively with cancer (or any health problem, for that matter). In any good drama, serendipity plays a role in the outcome, and at this point the first seemingly-serendipitous event in our journey occurred (more on this later). Our neighbor recommended an Oriental Medicine Doctor in Santa Monica. This turned out to be *the* life-changing moment for us, although we wouldn't realize it for many more weeks.

In the meantime, what was becoming clear is that conventional treatments are rarely a smart treatment choice. In the sections that follow, we share the "big picture" view of conventional cancer treatment that we developed through our research in 2002, and have refined and confirmed ever since.[15]

Conventional Cancer Treatment

When you go to see a conventional doctor about cancer, you are given only a very limited set of choices about treatment options, and only very harmful treatments at that. This information is presented to you as if it represents the entire spectrum of knowledge about how

---

15. Note that we go into much more detail in later chapters as to how we arrived at these conclusions.

to deal with cancer. *It does not.* And it's also presented to you along with all sorts of statistics that supposedly provide evidence to support the effectiveness of those treatments, and their appropriateness for you and your cancer. *They do not.*

When most doctors speak about cancer treatment, they are referring to four things: surgery, chemotherapy, radiation, and hormone therapy. Different surgical procedures may be available, and different drugs may be used for chemotherapy, but the approaches essentially are all the same. The cancer industry is very much an assembly line, and this is by design. There is a concept called the "standard of care" in medicine, and it's the process by which standard practices are established (and enforced) in medicine. On the surface, it sounds like a reasonable concept, but it's one that has run amuck when it comes to cancer care. The notion of a "standard of care" in cancer treatment, together with a host of other social and legal pressures, and with perverse profit incentives on the part of the pharmaceutical industry, has created an entire industry in lockstep, but moving in the wrong direction. The result is a narrow-minded, one-size-fits-all approach to cancer.

Surgery

Technically speaking, surgery is the best form of conventional treatment available, as it literally removes the cancer from one's body, allowing the body to recover more easily. However, we later learned that other schools of thought explain that surgery sometimes can "anger" the cancer, often causing a once relatively encapsulated cancer to be opened up, making it easier to spread. And because surgery is difficult on the body, it leaves the body weaker to defend against threats to it.

"In my opinion, the more surgical procedures (and accompanying disruptions to the immune system), the greater the risk of cancer spreading and manifesting in another location."[16]

"I believe that surgery can actually enhance the growth of systemic cancer because the removal of a tumor creates a tremendous amount of damage to healthy tissue and causes significant inflammation. Inflammation and the breakdown of tissue create an environment of very high free-radical activity in which cells are actively dividing in order to replace damaged cells, thus making it possible for an increase in the growth of the cancer itself. Postsurgical healing causes tremendous stress to the immune system, leading to systemic immune suppression that renders one vulnerable to a host of infections and/or more aggressive systemic cancer growth."[17]

For her part, Hollie now says that if she could do it all over again, she wouldn't have had her tumors removed surgically—the only conventional treatment she had—but instead would have enjoyed the empowering experience of watching traditional medical wisdom melt the lumps away.

Chemotherapy

The goal of chemotherapy is to reduce the risk of a systemic recurrence (i.e. having the cancer set up camp in other parts of the body). Chemotherapy has become a multi-billion dollar business.

---

16. Donald R. Yance, *Herbal Medicine, Healing & Cancer* (Chicago: Keats Publishing, 1999), 322-3.

17. Ibid., pp. 323-4.

For breast cancer in particular, but for most other cancers too, chemotherapy is a treatment approach in search of a justification for the billions of dollars and years of effort expended in trying to make it "work." All of this work has yielded mountains of studies and statistics that increasingly obscure the ineffectiveness of chemotherapy. Nearly all cancer statistics are bloated averages that have very little to do with unique individuals, and yet those numbers are communicated as if they were as unique to you as your fingerprints. Remember also that the guiding principle of the Hippocratic Oath is "First, do no harm." Chemotherapy goes against this principle, and one has to wonder if this has something to do with the disappearance of the Hippocratic Oath from modern medicine.

At the time of Hollie's diagnosis, our doctors gave us very firm advice that Hollie needed chemotherapy, radiation, and hormone therapy. They were wrong. They made a medical mistake, and we were barely lucky enough to catch the mistake in time. And it turns out this isn't uncommon. Doctors give women the wrong treatment for breast cancer about 90 percent of the time. With regard to breast cancer, for every 10 women who receive chemotherapy (and who have cancer similar to Hollie's), seven would have remained healthy without it, two would have had a recurrence anyway, and one would be spared a recurrence due to the chemotherapy. This means that in nine out of 10 cases, chemotherapy is either unnecessary or ineffective.[18,19]

That figure—90 percent of women incorrectly subjected to the

18. Reported by one of Hollie's oncologists in 2002.

19. Susan M. Love, M.D., "Doctors Rethink the Wisdom of Chemo for Breast-Cancer," *The Wall Street Journal*, October 8, 2002.

ravages of potentially deadly chemical treatments—is *not* being revealed in this book for the first time. It's widely known. But we actually weren't aware of this specific statistic when we made our decision to turn down chemotherapy. Our oncologist presented it to us *after* we explained to her that Hollie would not be undergoing chemotherapy. It was only then that she said she actually understood our decision, and presented us with this shocking statistic.

In her lymph nodes, Hollie had what is called micrometastasis. This means that there were microscopic cancer cells that had begun to spread to the lymph nodes. According to all the doctors, the mere presence of any cancer cells in the lymph nodes meant that the cancer was now in the circulatory system and could spread anywhere (i.e. metastasize to other parts of the body). And we agree with this point. We'll even go farther and point to the fact that on any given day, there are thousands of cancer cells present in the average person. "It is estimated that our normal cells in the course of cell division contain thousands of DNA errors, which are fortunately detected and repaired."[20] But Hollie's doctors believed that this was yet another signal that she needed aggressive chemotherapy and other harsh treatments. "The conclusion that chemotherapy is the only or best way to deal with these pockets of cancer (or that the micrometastases will necessarily turn into life-threatening cancer) is still speculative. In a sense, we can say that this approach stands on about as much solid ground as did the old Halsted radical mastectomy theory."[21]

---

20. Susan M. Love, M.D., *Dr. Susan Love's Breast Book, Third Edition, Fully Revised* (Cambridge: Perseus Publishing, 2000), 193-4.

21. SN Austin and C. Hitchcock, *Breast Cancer: What You Should Know (But May Not Be Told) About Prevention, Diagnosis and Treatment* (Rocklin: Prima, 1994).

Radiation

Radiation is aimed at reducing the chance of one having a local recurrence (i.e. having the cancer return to the original cancer site such as the breasts in the example of breast cancer). Following our decision not to move ahead with chemotherapy, we then took the next week or two to revisit our research about whether or not to have Hollie undergo radiation. The research about radiation actually is presented more straightforwardly, so the decision was fairly obvious to us. However, once again, we had to look for the research in order to determine this, as compared to just listening to what our doctors were telling us. In short, the research was very clear that while there sometimes was a reduction in *local recurrence* with radiation, there was no difference in *survival*. In other words, one was just as likely to be alive in five years if you did radiation, as compared to if you did not undergo radiation.

Hormone Therapy

Hormone therapy[22] drugs are used to treat hormone-sensitive cancers, and are essentially a way to "trick" cancer, both by reducing the amount of estrogen in the body, and also by blocking the effect of estrogen on estrogen-sensitive cells (also called estrogen receptor positive, or ER+ cancers).[23] The research on hormone therapy is as unflattering as that of any conventional treatment. Many studies

---

22. Hormone therapy is entirely unrelated to the harmful hormone replacement therapy (HRT) that became popular with conventional physicians in the 1990s, and which was eventually found to *cause* cancer. http://www.breastcancer.org/treatment/hormonal/.

23. http://www.breastcancer.org/treatment/hormonal/.

show that it actually creates a *worse* prognosis for the women taking it, and in addition to failing to work on the primary cancer for which it's diagnosed, one side effect of one of the more common drugs is a substantially increased risk of secondary cancers, such as endometrial cancer.[24] As we discuss in Chapter 7, had we not rejected conventional treatments, Hollie would very likely have had a cancer recurrence as a direct result of taking Tamoxifen, a common hormone therapy drug used to treat breast cancer.

We Can Do Better

After a broad and deep consideration of the treatments being presented to us as urgent and essential by conventional oncology, we were left with an overwhelming feeling of, "Is this as good as it gets?" As we were soon to find out, the answer is a resounding "No." It soon got *much* better for us.

---

24. Susan M. Love, M.D., *Dr. Susan Love's Breast Book, Third Edition, Fully Revised* (Cambridge: Perseus Publishing, 2000), 393.

CHAPTER SIX

Decision

"In a last-minute twist, you decided to go another route...and not just any route, a very unconventional route that would change your life forever."

—FRIEND

"Hollie, you *need* chemotherapy." We still remember those words as clearly as any we can recall from our experience. This exact quote came from an immensely smart, kind, and well-meaning oncologist in Los Angeles, but, all of the oncologists with whom we were dealing were saying the exact same thing—Hollie needed intense chemotherapy, radiation, possibly some additional surgery,[25] and at least five years of hormone therapy. It wasn't optional. It was necessary to prevent what they all agreed was a very aggressive cancer from coming back, all over her body, and killing her.

We have to admit, it was compelling. And the social pressure to conform was intense. It turns out that all the patients suffering from cancer have copied the lockstep approach of their doctors. Virtually everyone we spoke to—friends, family, survivors—had already frozen their minds on "getting through it." But to us, none of it was making

---

25. This was the only detail—the need for additional surgery—about which there was any variation of opinion amongst our doctors.

any sense. We knew that none of these treatments did anything to address the underlying factors that allowed Hollie's cancer to develop in the first place. This was becoming more clear to us by the day, especially in light of our ever-expanding reading about traditional medical wisdom, and how it was being combined with the very latest science available to offer a much smarter, much safer approach to dealing with cancer. But again, this was all still very new to us, and we still hadn't yet found a comprehensive strategy for what to do in lieu of any conventional treatment. It seemed like we were going to have to go to war, but not because "diplomacy" with our cancer had failed. Rather, we had to start the killing simply because we hadn't yet figured out a way to make peace with our cancer.

But we were close.

Saturday, September 14, 2002

Like most people dutifully suffering through chemotherapy, as we were resigning ourselves to the fact that we were going to have to accept it as our only option, we nonetheless were going to do so our way, with humor and determination. One example was the rationalization that chemotherapy, radiation, and hormone therapy wouldn't be as bad as the treatment preferred by Hollie's mother—who humorously-but-understandably wanted a swift "torso-ectomy" to get rid of any chance of cancer coming back. We had this mental image of Hollie spending the rest of her life as just a head attached to a pair of legs!

In another example, with Hollie's first chemotherapy treatment less than three weeks away, we asked a close friend of ours to host a "chemo-kick off party" for us. The purpose of the party was to thank all of our friends for the love and support they had provided, and to show that we would meet the challenge head on, and with good cheer. We asked everyone to cover their hair in creative ways—hats, wigs, etc. And because Hollie was actually about to lose her hair, she was the only person who did not have to wear anything on her head. It was one of those moments of incredible love and support that you hear about in most cancer stories. And everybody left the party that evening thinking they had become part of another cancer saga, and so did we. But this was about to become anything but just another cancer tale.

Wednesday, September 25, 2002

It was now less than a week before Hollie was scheduled to show up at the chemotherapy lab, and to welcome an intravenous needle into her arm with a payload that would destroy nearly every dividing cell in her body, all in the name of health. We struggled more than ever with the logical absurdity of it all.

On this day we had an appointment with an Oriental Medicine Doctor (OMD). At the time, she was not a primary cancer care specialist, and thus her role was going to be supportive. She was going to do the best she could with Chinese medicine and related wisdom to try to protect the body from the damaging treatments, and to help it heal as quickly and completely as possible afterwards. Her office was like a spa. So serene, and so unlike any of the other doctors' offices we had been visiting. At the end of our appointment, she whirled around in her office chair to face some bookshelves behind her desk. "One last thing," she said. She pulled a book from the shelf, and recommended that we read it—*Herbal Medicine, Healing, and Cancer*, by Donald Yance, a renowned herbalist.

And in that moment, our neighbor had cured Hollie's cancer. Our neighbor sent us to the OMD, who pulled that book off the shelf. And that was it. It was the scientific *and* safe approach that we'd been craving. Despite being fairly technically dense, we read the entire book that evening. With every turn of the page, the world was making sense again! The multi-pathway efficacy of botanical medicine! The synergistic effects on cancer of multiple natural compounds working in concert! Nutritional science as the cornerstone of cancer-free living! And all of it *deeply* scientific (the book had nearly 500 citations, many of which dovetailed with the intense research we'd been conducting), and built on a foundation of health and healing for the body.

The author had a clinic in Oregon called The Centre for Natural Healing (CNH). We called first thing the next morning.

Thursday, September 26, 2002

The first appointment that Hollie could get with a CNH practitioner was for October 30 (which was nearly six weeks away). We took the appointment with a senior practitioner and began filling out the required paperwork, including an extensive medical history, and sending over Hollie's medical records. But this would be well after the start of Hollie's conventional treatment. Again, we resigned ourselves to the fact that whatever wisdom we'd be able to glean from traditional medicine would have to be supplementary, and also a way to restore as much damaged body functioning from the treatments as we could. That's how the typical cancer story would unfold. But this wasn't just another cancer story.

Friday, September 27, 2002

Hollie received a call from her oncologist's office. She was due to begin chemotherapy the following Monday, September 30, but the office had a scheduling conflict. They rescheduled her for Wednesday, October 2. It was nothing short of a stay of execution for Hollie's immune system.

Monday, September 30, 2002

We received a call from CNH saying that they, too, had had a schedule change. But this one was a cancellation, which created an opening for an initial consultation the next day, Tuesday, October 1, just one day before the *rescheduled* chemotherapy was to begin! We took the new appointment with tremendous enthusiasm, but we still weren't fully aware of what was unfolding, and at the very last possible moment.

Tuesday, October 1, 2002

Hollie had now begun taking steroids in order to prepare her body for the massive damage the chemotherapy would begin to cause in one more day. (This is one of the many topics that "just come up," nonchalantly, as you're discussing and preparing for cancer treatment.) Upon taking the steroids, she immediately began suffering from severe leg pain during the day and especially at night, which was dismissed by her then-primary oncologist in charge of overseeing Hollie's treatment. Hollie was losing sleep already, and yet hadn't even had her first drop of poison.

Later that afternoon, we had our conference call with CNH. The two-hour consultation was the most in-depth discussion of cancer we'd ever had, bar none. It wasn't even close. At the end of our call, our practitioner calmly but firmly recommended that we postpone chemotherapy for just one week, in order to allow CNH time to thoroughly review our case. We hung up the phone, only to pick it up a few seconds later to speed dial the chemotherapy lab to postpone the first treatment.

"Would you like to reschedule now?"

"No, thank you. We'll call back to reschedule."

It's nearly eight years later as we write this, and we have yet to call back.

Sunday, October 6, 2002

The clinic spent several days reviewing Hollie's case collaboratively (similar to the "tumor boards" that transpire in most oncology offices), and with a very close look at Hollie's individual characteristics and traits—of her body, her cancer, and more. That Sunday, we received written treatment recommendations from our CNH practitioner. The message was clear, confident, and logical—they were strongly recommending that we postpone conventional treatment for at least three months (and possibly indefinitely), in favor of an aggressive herbal treatment protocol, combined with very close monitoring, and together with recommendations about detoxifying our diet and overall lifestyle. Their reasoning was matter-of-fact. The conventional doctors were foisting upon us a one-size-fits-all, overly aggressive and harmful treatment plan that had little chance of doing anything other than making Hollie very sick, and possibly making her cancer much worse. Only later would we learn just how disastrous a mistake the conventional treatments would have been (see the "No Strength in These Numbers: Hormone Therapy" section of chapter 7). By now, however, we were finally moving in a safer direction, very much leaning in the direction of traditional medicine. We had found a comprehensive plan that was as aggressive as it was comprehensive, but still safe.

All that remained at this point was for us to decide formally. All that remained was for us to look the world of conventional cancer treatment in the eye, and say, "No, we've found a better way."

Tuesday, October 8, 2002

Though we'd finally identified an approach to cancer that was smarter and safer than the conventional treatments being offered, we were nonetheless still frozen. Time stopped for us over the next couple of days after receiving the 14-page return-to-health protocol from the clinic. It was all there—more than 70 pills per day, teas, tinctures, smoothies with all manner of powders and other compounds, and so much more, all upon a foundation of total lifestyle transformation, from personal care products to exercise regimen to spiritual life, and everything in between. But still we paused. We talked essentially non-stop from Sunday to Monday. On Monday, we took a long walk in beautiful Palisades Park in Santa Monica, perched above the beaches of Santa Monica Bay, and overlooking the Pacific Ocean. The response that we thought everyone, especially the doctors, would have to our decision was palpable. And now you know how Hollie came up with the title of this book.

"You did *what*?!!"

"Who turns down her doctor's advice? In the 21st century, in a major U.S. city like Los Angeles? When you're *twenty seven*? And you have *cancer*??!!"

But an even heavier weight than that of social pressure was the crushing load of this question, which Hollie turned to Patrick and asked, as the sun was setting on the horizon that day.

"What if I do this natural medicine thing, and the cancer comes back? And what if I die?"

And that's when we knew we were on to something. That's when we knew that we'd done our homework, and we were seeing the entire truth. When you can see the full truth about something, then one side of it can't become all-consuming, and in particular all-consumingly frightening. The full truth about modern cancer treatment yields the following response, which immediately defangs the beast that was Hollie's question. One of our close family friends had helped us along towards this realization, when she responded calmly to the, "What if we don't do conventional treatment, and we're wrong?" question by asking, "But what if you do, and you're wrong?" Patrick looked into Hollie's eyes, and reminded her of these wise words, "But what if you do conventional treatment, and everything we now know about it turns out to be true for you, and the cancer gets worse, and you die?"

In that moment, Hollie officially decided to hold off indefinitely on conventional treatments, and proceed full-speed ahead with the aggressive herbal medicine treatment protocol recommended by CNH.

It was one of those quintessential moments of divine clarity. That afternoon, Hollie found a state of calm confidence amidst the fear, complexity, and pressure, and she gave herself over to the wisdom of Mother Nature, and to the combined wisdom of 5,000[26] years of eclectic and effective traditional medicine, integrated prudently with modern science. The view from Palisades Park was postcard-beautiful, and that's pretty much exactly how we felt about the decision that day, and ever since.

It should be noted that while Patrick was an incredible pillar of strength and support to Hollie, he *never once* told her what he thought she should do. He knew better than to do that, since one of Hollie's primary struggles was feeling trapped, like she had no choice over what was going to happen to her body and life. Patrick knew that if he gave an unsolicited opinion one way or another, he would be "one of them"—just another voice pressuring her to conform to a treatment approach.

Despite flying high about the decision, we felt a responsibility to try to convey to our friends, family, and doctors that we hadn't made it lightly. Not in the least. So we crafted a "Treatment Decision" document and sent it around to everyone we knew (see Appendix A for a copy of the original document). In response, we received an email from that dear friend who had organized the "chemo-kick off

---

26. We use "5,000 years" throughout the book to refer to the oldest healing traditions and wisdom on record. Ayurveda, Chinese medicine, and herbal medicine from ancient Sumeria all date this far back in history. http://en.wikipedia.org/wiki/Traditional_medicine.

party." It still remains one of our most cherished and deepest belly-laughs of the entire experience.

"After the greatest potluck party in the whole world, this is how you decide to repay me?!? With a slap in the face! Well, SOMEBODY is getting chemo, even if it has to be ME!"

CHAPTER SEVEN

Proof or Spoof? The Case Against Conventional Cancer Treatment

"Hollie and Patrick did what not many people would do—
they immersed themselves into research about breast cancer,
treatments, different types of chemo and what their side effects
were...not being able to enjoy fully the birth of their daughter."

—FRIEND

We are not anti-Western medicine. In fact, what we learned via our journey is a deep appreciation for the areas where Western medicine is indeed seemingly miraculous. But along with that we also came face-to-face with its very definite limits. Conventional medicine is very good at dealing with structural problems, and it achieves this success via truly stunning advances in diagnostic technology and surgical precision. If you're in a serious car accident, traditional medicine isn't going to help you. Emergency medicine will. If you blow out your knee, all the botanical science in the world isn't going to repair that. An expert surgeon will, and in addition he/she will probably have you on your feet in days or perhaps even hours. But for systemic, chronic disease, conventional medicine is a sub-standard form of medical care.

As a friend asked in the quote at the beginning of our opening chapter, why would a young woman with cancer, surrounded by 21st century medical experts in a major American metropolis, and with everything to lose, choose to reject the advice of her doctors to follow the prescribed conventional treatment for cancer? Our answer to that is simple: Conventional cancer treatment simply didn't make sense to us. In our view, the logic underlying it was (and remains) fundamentally and irreparably flawed. Scientific research made a very weak case for it. Questionable ethics further undercut its credibility. And, finally, a thick layer of media bias led us to realize that most people follow conventional treatments, not because they really want to, or because they're convinced of their effectiveness, but rather because most of the information we discovered through our journey is pretty well hidden from view. The healing path cannot easily be seen from the main road.

The Tortured Logic of Conventional Cancer Treatment

The first thing that gave us pause as we evaluated the treatments being offered by our conventional doctors was the illogic of it all. Cancer is fundamentally a failure of the functioning of the immune system, and conventional cancer treatments are disastrously damaging to that very immune system. Chemotherapy drugs and radiation are themselves carcinogenic. Even surgery is deeply immunosuppressive. So the logic of conventional cancer treatment holds that it's sensible to destroy the body on the theory that doing so is at least destroying the cancer as well. This is the medical equivalent of carpet bombing a city during wartime. As Dr. Andrew Weil suggested, it's nothing short of medieval thinking, at best.

Where's the Science?

In addition to struggling with the illogic of conventional treatments, we next embarked upon a close look at the scientific research behind the treatments being recommended. The most common retort we got from medical doctors whenever we brought up traditional therapies of any kind was an immediate "That's not science!" We found exactly the opposite to be true, however. The traditional healing systems and philosophies we researched were deeply scientific, especially the one employed by the clinic that treated Hollie. They also tended to be highly individualized. By contrast, we discovered that virtually all of the research recommending conventional treatments failed to hold up under scrutiny. The only blind faith we discovered on our journey was an almost cultish devotion, on the part of the medical establishment, to the so-called "science" that is supposed to underly conventional medicine. Conventional cancer research has become a "fiefdom of expertise,"[27] one in which scientific thinking that is deep and broad, and ever-cognizant of the human bodies involved, is nowhere to be found. The result of this is that conventional cancer treatment is very much a one-size-fits-all approach. Worse, there are mountains of research showing quite plainly that conventional treatments are ineffective

---

27. John Ralston Saul, *Voltaire's Bastards* (New York: Vintage Books, 1992), 8. Saul's book is an excellent foray into what's wrong with much modern medical research. "The reality is that the division of knowledge into feudal fiefdoms of expertise has made general understanding and coordinated action not simply impossible, but despised and distrusted." It would be hard to find a more apt description of modern conventional cancer treatment.

and harmful.

Also, in looking back now, knowing what we know, it's hard to put into words the breathtaking arrogance of pushing aside nearly 5,000 years of accumulated medical wisdom, and replacing it with the narrow-minded "modern science" of the past few decades. Is there anything *less* scientific than this kind of approach?

No Strength in These Numbers: Chemotherapy

Since chemotherapy was being recommended so strenuously to Hollie, our natural inclination was to ask why. Surely there would be a clear justification for subjecting a 28 year-old woman to devastating treatments that themselves would cause some number of the following health problems: dangerously low white blood cell counts, severe nausea and vomiting, diarrhea, burning or tingling in the extremities, dangerously low platelet counts, mouth sores, sores in the digestive tract, changes in heart rhythm, high or low blood pressure, blood in the stool, severe fluid retention, difficulty breathing, rashes, decreased bone marrow function, extreme fatigue, easy bruising or bleeding, congestive heart failure, irregular heartbeats, liver damage, seizures, early menopause/sterility, secondary cancers, and many other ailments related to or caused by these common side effects.[28] Some of these would be permanent. Others would linger for many years to come. There is even the risk of death itself as a result of the damage caused by conventional cancer treatments. And these are just the physical ramifications. Oncology nurses will tell you there's

---

28. This list is comprised of just *some* of the known side effects from the specific chemotherapy drugs prescribed to Hollie.

little or no quality of life for those undergoing these treatments. For subjecting Hollie to all that, we should be guaranteed never to hear from cancer again, right? Wrong. *Very* wrong.

The "benefit" of chemotherapy for Hollie was described as follows: If she followed the treatments prescribed by her medical doctors, she had an 80 percent chance of never hearing from cancer again. And if she did nothing at all? Surely her odds of having to grapple with a perhaps much more serious cancer would shoot through the roof without the benefits of 21st century conventional cancer treatment, right? Wrong. If Hollie did *nothing* at all following the lump removal, she still had a whopping 70 percent chance of never hearing from cancer again. *Huh?* A 10 percent improvement in the odds of having a recurrence of her cancer? In exchange for *five years* of harmful treatments? So then our minds immediately zeroed in on that 10 percent improvement figure. What exactly did it mean for a person to have a 10 percent lower chance of having a recurrence? Did that mean Hollie's immune system would be 10 percent stronger than before, thus making it 10 percent stronger to fend off a return of her cancer? Certainly not. Chemotherapy devastates the body, and the immune system in particular, and it takes years to recover from it, and most people never *fully* recover. Did it mean she'd have a 10 percent extension of cancer-free living tacked on to the end of her life?

These questions were never answered for us, and that's because they can't be answered. The reality is that cancer statistics are largely meaningless to individuals. And honest physicians will admit to this. Dr. Susan Love, in her *Breast Book*, describes the sad state of cancer statistics:

"Unfortunately we are left guessing on the basis of probabilities that are not individualized. This usually means that we overtreat, fearing that we might miss someone who could benefit."[29]

Once again, the statistics that you hear in the doctor's office have little if anything to do with you, your life, your body, and your cancer. And beyond the fact that these numbers consist largely of averages, probabilities, and guesswork, the numbers and other information you hear from a medical doctor may simply be wrong. Studies show that doctors routinely overestimate the benefits of treatment when communicating with patients. One study showed that doctors thought the benefits of chemotherapy were *three times better than they actually were.*[30]

So there we were, trying to get our heads around the meaning of this 10 percent reduced risk of a recurrence, weighed against the tremendous toll of the chemotherapy. So we pushed ahead, researching even more deeply the language doctors use to sell chemotherapy. All the while, Dr. Susan Love's words about guesswork, averages, and probabilities were echoing in our heads. The more we learned, the less convincing it all became.

Overstating Benefits and Understating Failures

Numerous studies have demonstrated how physicians routinely overstate the benefits of conventional treatments, while at the same

29. Susan M. Love, M.D., *Dr. Susan Love's Breast Book, Third Edition, Fully Revised* (Cambridge: Perseus Publishing, 2000), 388.

30. S. Rajagopal, PJ Goodman and IF Tannock, "Adjuvant Chemotherapy for Breast Cancer: Discordance Between physicians' perception of Benefit and the Results of Clinical Trials," *Journal of Clinical Oncology* 12, no. 6 (1994): 1296.

time understating the failures, and in particular minimizing the damage caused by the treatments. For example, the *Journal of Clinical Oncology* reports that "oncologists' perceptions of the results of clinical trials overestimate the therapeutic gain from use of adjuvant chemotherapy for breast cancer."[31] The rush to "help" has created a clear pattern of dishonesty in the cancer industry.

"Many people with cancer of the pancreas...receive some form of chemotherapy...Remarkably, there is no evidence that the procedure can either cure the disease or extend life for the person who has it. In fact, the opposite seems to be the case. In one study, published in the journal *Cancer*, the median survival for untreated patients after diagnosis was 3.9 months. For those who received chemotherapy, however, the median survival was 3.0 months."[32]

Patients who underwent chemotherapy actually died *sooner.*

"A 1989 report from the U.S. General Accounting Office found no increase in longevity for premenopausal women who chose chemotherapy—as opposed to those who did not—as a treatment for Stage II (or earlier) breast cancers. Nor did chemotherapy improve survival for node-positive postmenopausal women."[33]

For breast cancer in particular, but for most cancers generally, the so-called "benefits" of chemotherapy are marginal, if they exist at all. If conventional physicians are routinely overstating benefits and understating failure, then this makes a bad situation even worse.

---

31. Ibid.

32. C. Frey et al., "Randomized Study of 5-FU and CCNU in Pancreatic Cancer," *Cancer* 47 (1981): 27-31.

33. Susun Weed, *Breast Cancer, Breast Health!* (Woodstock: Ash Tree Publishing, 1996), 227.

Doctor-Patient Communication

Understandably, conventional physicians are eager to provide some good news to patients, especially as they're faced with the unforgiving task of having to administer such harmful treatments to their patients. Unfortunately, this exacerbates the problem of doctors having a skewed recall of information from studies, such that much information communicated from doctor to patient is simply factually incorrect. Dr. Susan Love recounts a typical example:

"Recently a woman called me for my advice. She…had been told by her oncologist that she should be on chemotherapy because her chance of dying in the next five years was 15 percent without chemotherapy. So she thought she might try it. I asked her if the doctor had told her what her chance of dying in the next five years was if she *did* [emphasis added] take chemo. He hadn't. "I assume it means I have a 100 percent chance of surviving the next five years if I take it," she said. I told her that wasn't accurate: her chance of dying with chemo was 13 percent."[34]

We have heard dozens of these types of communication failures between doctor and patient over the years, regarding not just cancer but various other medical conditions as well. But with cancer, the fear instilled by the diagnosis and the severity of treatment being directed at you cripples most people from asking all the clarifying questions that need to be asked. Properly understanding the answers is a bigger challenge still. Our experiences since Hollie's diagnosis tell us that virtually all cancer patients misunderstand these numbers, which

---

34. Susan M. Love, M.D., *Dr. Susan Love's Breast Book, Third Edition, Fully Revised* (Cambridge: Perseus Publishing, 2000), 381.

leads to poorly understood treatment decisions, and ultimately, to medical mistakes.

In our view, there isn't enough honesty from the medical establishment about just how harmful conventional cancer treatment is, especially when considering how unnecessary and/or ineffective it is in so many cases. And there's nearly total silence from the conventional cancer business about the wide variety of ways in which people cure cancer all the time without subjecting themselves to harmful, ineffective conventional treatments. In Hollie's case, a good example of this was that, on the one hand, her oncologists told her that the side effects of chemotherapy wouldn't be "that bad." Yet, she was also told to avoid going to public places, because her immune system would be so crippled as to be vulnerable to even basic infections. In addition, there was a clear gap between the information we were reading ourselves about the damage caused by chemotherapy, and what we were being told by our doctors. And when Hollie spoke to actual cancer patients undergoing conventional treatments, the truth was even more acute. The most upbeat of the patients described "good days and bad days," with a heavy gravity of tone about the latter, as if trying to communicate a secret message. Others were more direct, reporting being in so much pain at times that all they could do is lay on the floor and cry.

A recent and personal example reminds us that this problem is still a very real and disturbing one for conventional cancer specialists. A family member of Hollie's with recurrent breast cancer was told by her doctor that a new chemotherapy drug being recommended "had one side effect; just some burning and dryness in the hands and feet." Some quick investigation into the drug revealed many other serious side effects. And this "mild irritation" described by the doctor about the hands and feet actually is termed "hand-foot syndrome," and it consists of "numbness, tingling, pain, redness, or blistering of the palms of the hands and soles of the feet. This can lead to the disappearance of fingerprints in some patients."[35] As a final insult, the drug also happened to be proven ineffective for this family member, as she'd had a round of chemotherapy that targeted cancer in the same way this new proposed drug did, but her cancer came back, worse (she had not gotten chemo-sensitivity testing[36]).

Statistical Tricks

As the hasty urge to help has combined with other developments in cancer treatment, in particular much-earlier diagnoses, various statistical tricks have found their way into information about cancer treatment, incidence, survival, and so forth.

"Chemotherapy practitioners do not want to think that the weapons they employ to kill cancer cells are of little or no use to their patients. They want to believe they are helping people, and in their defense they point to the substantial increases in the "five-year-survival" rates for many cancers that have occurred during the years of chemotherapy use. Unfortunately, these improvements have been

---

35. http://en.wikipedia.org/wiki/Capecitabine. For a report on the disappearance of fingerprints specifically, see http://www.usnews.com/health/family-health/cancer/articles/2009/05/27/fingerprints-may-vanish-with-cancer-drug.html.

36. Chemotherapy sensitivity testing entails matching one's actual cancer cells (taken from a biopsy) with multiple chemotherapy drugs in order to identify which drugs will be *effective*, and which drugs will be *ineffective*. We discuss this topic in detail later in the book.

repeatedly shown to be mainly statistical artifacts. Thanks to new, sophisticated diagnostic techniques (MRIs, CAT scans, biochemical and DNA markers), and more widespread screening for cancer (mammograms, PSA tests for prostate cancer, Pap smears, etc.), many cancers are discovered today much earlier than they used to be. Thus the meter that measures "five-year survival" from time of diagnosis starts running sooner."[37]

In addition, we learned that cancer mortality statistics are obtained from The National Center for Health Statistics (NCHS), which is part of the Centers for Disease Control (CDC). According to a health statistician there with whom we spoke, each patient's doctor is responsible for writing the "immediate cause of death" on the death certificate. If there were two or more conditions involved, then it's the doctor's discretion as to which one was the official (primary) cause of death. This means that when cancer patients undergoing treatment die from the treatment itself (pneumonia, heart or other organ failure, fatal infections, etc.), or die years later from side effects of treatments, are we to believe that "cancer" will reliably and consistently be listed as the immediate cause of death? The doctor to whom we spoke at the NCHS confirmed that there is no formal system or protocol for categorizing a death as caused by cancer versus, say, heart failure from a chemo drug used to treat the cancer. Given the marginal benefits of conventional cancer treatments presented by formal research, if even just a small percentage of all death certificates improperly attribute the "immediate cause of death" to be something other than cancer, then official survival rates would change significantly.

---

37. John Robbins, *Reclaiming Our Health* (Tiburon: HJ Kramer, 1998), 240.

Recurrence versus Survival

We've noticed that most doctors routinely move back and forth between talking about recurrence versus survival. Granted, recurrent cancer is generally more serious than when you're first diagnosed. But getting caught up in discussing recurrence instead of survival is a good way to get confused about the true value of your treatment options. We observed that statistics showing improvement in recurrence rates are more often communicated by doctors. But if you reduce your recurrence risk, yet your survival risk stays the same, what have you really gained? Patients are only concerned with survival. Of what value is any other benefit to you, besides survival, other than to know that you're providing statistical fodder for conventional treatments?

Cure versus Benefit or Response

A variation on the confusion of the terms "recurrence" and "survival" is the same misuse of "cure" versus "benefit" or "response." You'll very commonly hear medical doctors speak with great confidence about the number of women who "benefit" from chemotherapy, or whose cancer will "respond" to the drugs. But again, these measures are all a distant second to survival. As one researcher aptly describes this problem, "If you can shrink the tumor 50 percent or more for 28 days, you have got the FDA's definition of an active drug. That is called a response rate, so you have a response... [but] when you look to see if there is any life prolongation from taking this treatment what you find is all kinds of hocus pocus and song and dance about the disease-free survival, and this and that."[38]

A related problem has to do with the very nature of conventional research itself. In virtually all studies, chemotherapy drugs are compared against *other* chemotherapy drugs. Over time, innovation has admittedly lowered the toxicity of the drugs being used. But this creates the deceptive impression that the drugs are improving all the time, when in reality they're primarily only improving relative to their more harmful predecessors. Furthermore, there is virtually zero research into people like Hollie, who eschew conventional treatments entirely, and who thus form the best possible control group. The lack of attention paid to such people by conventional research is a troubling blind spot in the so-called science behind conventional cancer treatments.

Relative versus Absolute Statistics

Probably the worst errors made by doctors in selling chemotherapy is talking about relative versus absolute benefits. If you have an 8 percent risk of having a cancer recurrence, and chemotherapy reduces that risk to 4 percent, that's a 4 percent absolute improvement in your risk, but it's a 50 percent relative improvement in your risk (4 is half, or 50 percent, of 8). Again, these risk factors are derived from large groups of patients being studied. They are statistical probabilities that are *not* individualized to you. Beware of doctors talking about large, double-digit benefits to doing chemotherapy. Numbers that are so obviously positive virtually never

---

38. Ralph Moss, Ph.D., "On Chemotherapy, Laetrile, Coley's Toxins, Burzynski, & Cancer Politics," *Laura Lee Radio Show*, 1994, http://www.alternative-doctor.com/cancer/mossinterview.htm.

exist for conventional cancer treatment.

Me or We?

And remember, the most honest conventional doctors will tell you that they simply don't know who will do poorly with cancer and who will be fine. *They don't know which individuals will win out over cancer and which ones will lose.* The research being done on conventional cancer treatments is a mad dash to find some criteria by which they can know who to treat, and how. So by definition, all cancer statistics are guesses. Educated ones, in a limited sense, but still guesses in the end. And this guessing leads to a vast amount of medical mistakes in the rush to "do something," and to try to establish some credibility for chemotherapy:

"Most women with breast cancer endure the agony of chemotherapy to improve their chance of survival. But the truth is, most of them would do just as well without it."[39]

Timing is Everything

Another troubling trend is the fact that the cancer studies being cited by doctors to sell chemotherapy are either outdated or based on too-short a period of time for the results to be relevant. If you look at the history of chemotherapy, the criticisms of it were much harsher in the 1980s and earlier. Criticisms from those periods typically went like this one, by Dr. Alan Levin of UCSF Medical School:

"Most cancer patients in this country die of chemotherapy. Chemotherapy does not eliminate breast, colon, or lung cancers. The

---

39. Susan M. Love, M.D., "Doctors Rethink the Wisdom of Chemo for Breast-Cancer," *The Wall Street Journal*, October 8, 2002.

fact has been documented for over a decade [that] women with breast cancer are likely to die faster with chemotherapy than without it."[40]

In the 1990s, the worst of the chemotherapy drugs began to get replaced by admittedly more sophisticated, less toxic mixtures. This had the benefit of ridding the world of the most deadly treatments, but it also meant that now we were using drugs that were still highly toxic, and for which there wasn't any long-term research about survival, damage from the drugs, and so forth. As an example, one of the drugs that had been prescribed to Hollie (Adriamycin) was requested to be withdrawn from use just a few years later, due to years upon years of documented "cardiac risks and increased risks of leukemias and other cancers associated with this drug."[41] (Note that, despite this study, Adriamycin is still widely used.)

Chemotherapy: The Big Picture

There are indeed some very clear but also very limited benefits to chemotherapy. Improvements in survival that are significant enough to justify the toxicity of chemotherapy are limited to only a few, usually rare cancers: "Chemotherapy is not an effective weapon against the vast majority of solid carcinomas in adults. It rarely extends overall survival, and the little advantage that may be gained is offset by the toxicity it generally causes...[However], there are situations where chemotherapy can be a rational and life-saving course. These include most cases of Hodgkin's disease, acute lymphocytic leukemia (ALL), and testicular cancer, as well as certain rare cancers, such as Burkitt's

---

40. http://www.ihealthtube.com/aspx/article.aspx?id=2368.

41. http://www.breastcancer.org/treatment/chemotherapy/new_research/20071213b. jsp.

lymphoma, choriocarcinoma, and lymphosarcoma...Basically, some chemotherapy has its uses...However, even for the above cancers, chemotherapy remains an often grueling option—medieval, by many doctors' own admission."[42]

We would argue that, even for the few cancers for which chemotherapy makes a significant-enough difference to justify the damage it causes, it may well still not be the best choice. Chemotherapy does nothing to address the underlying causes of cancer, and thus even for the rare cancers that "respond" to it significantly, there are more prudent treatment options to consider.

Although it wasn't available until after we'd made our decision to reject conventional cancer treatment, a major study published in 2004 documented what we had concluded two years earlier. Namely, that there just isn't a good scientific case for subjecting oneself to the ravages of chemotherapy. The study investigated the contribution of chemotherapy to five-year survival rates with 22 major adult malignancies, and it showed startling results. Dr. Ralph Moss[43] expands on this recent and important study as follows:

"[A]ll three of the paper's authors are oncologists. Their meticulous study was based on an analysis of the results of all the

---

42. Ralph W. Moss, Ph.D., *Questioning Chemotherapy* (Brooklyn: Equinox Press, 2000), 8.

43. Ralph W. Moss, Ph.D. has spent decades investigating and writing about cancer. Formerly the assistant director of public affairs at Memorial Sloan-Kettering Cancer Center, Dr. Moss is the author of such groundbreaking books as *Cancer Therapy*, *Questioning Chemotherapy*, and *The Cancer Industry*, as well as the award-winning PBS documentary "The Cancer War." Dr. Moss was a founding advisor to the National Institutes of Health's Office of Alternative Medicine, and is presently scientific advisor to the Rosenthal Center of Columbia University and the University of Texas School of Public Health.

randomized, controlled clinical trials (RCTs) performed in Australia and the U.S. that reported a statistically significant increase in 5-year survival due to the use of chemotherapy in adult malignancies. Survival data were drawn from the Australian cancer registries and the U.S. National Cancer Institute's Surveillance Epidemiology and End Results (SEER) registry spanning the period January 1990 until January 2004. Wherever data were uncertain, the authors deliberately erred on the side of over-estimating the benefit of chemotherapy. Even so, the study concluded that overall, chemotherapy contributes just over 2 percent to improved survival in cancer patients. Yet despite the mounting evidence of chemotherapy's lack of effectiveness in prolonging survival, oncologists continue to present chemotherapy as a rational and promising approach to cancer treatment."[44]

Please read those results again. A 21st century study has shown that the survival of a mere two percent of cancer patients overall is improved by chemotherapy. This study got virtually zero coverage in the American media, but it didn't escape the glare of best-selling economists Steven Levitt and Stephen Dubner, who report on the research in their book, *SuperFreakonomics*:

"An exhaustive analysis of cancer treatment in the United States and Australia showed that the five-year survival rate for all patients was about 63 percent but that chemotherapy contributed barely 2 percent to this result. There is a long list of cancers for which chemotherapy has *zero* discernible effect."[45]

---

44. Ralph W. Moss, Ph.D., "Aussie Oncologists Criticize Chemotherapy–Part One," March 5, 2006, http://www.cancerdecisions.com/030506.html.

45. Steven D. Levitt and Stephen J. Dubner, *SuperFreakonomics* (New York: William Morrow, 2009), 84.

As one reviewer summarized, "They might have gone a step further and said, 'Overall, prayer is better than chemo. At least prayer causes no pain.'"[46]

No Strength in These Numbers: Radiation

As we tussled with our conventional doctors over the vast amount of information we were finding that indicated chemotherapy was not a smart choice for Hollie's cancer, we next moved to reviewing the case for radiation, which was also being recommended for Hollie. On the surface, radiation seemed to us to be less damaging to the body than chemotherapy, but this isn't actually true.

Our research led us to believe that in the event of a local recurrence, the possibility of additional surgery was *much easier* on the body compared to radiation, a known carcinogen. As articulated in Hollie's herbal oncology treatment recommendations, "aside from the damage radiation does to healthy cells, and the failure to increase survival time, it does not do anything to actually change the underlying constitution that allowed cancer to develop in the first place. If cancer is going to recur, then it is best that [it] comes back in the breast where it is not going to complicate other organs, where it is accessible to surgery, and where there are still other chemotherapy agents to try. It is much worse when cancer recurs in the bone or liver or brain, which is where breast cancer secondaries tend to go. In summary, without radiation, a recurrence if it does occur, will most likely be in the breast, whereas with radiation, secondaries could be driven from the breast to other tissues which could then be more

---

46. http://econlog.econlib.org/archives/2009/10/the_high_points.html.

complicated to manage."[47]

In one of those moments that came to symbolize our cancer journey, we were in the office of the conventional oncologist we'd chosen to oversee Hollie's monitoring, discussing treatment options. She had finally relented on our insistence that chemotherapy seemed like an exceedingly poor choice. "But," she said, "I really want you to do a course of radiation to make sure the cancer doesn't come back locally." By then, she knew better than not to have research ready to support her recommendation, so she had one of her thick medical texts open to a table showing a clear reduction in the return of cancer in the breast following radiation treatment. The results were neatly organized in a table on the page. Hollie looked at the page, by now knowing exactly what she was looking for, lifted the book into her hands, and pointed to another neatly-organized table of data, this time about the survival of women who'd gotten radiation treatment, versus those who had not. The difference?

Zero.

In many ways, the research about radiation showed that it was an even poorer choice than chemotherapy. Below is a brief listing of the kinds of typical, damning findings we discovered in regard to radiation:

- "[T]here were no definite differences in overall survival at 10 years."[48]

---

47. Hollie's herbal oncology treatment recommendations, Centre for Natural Healing, 2002.

48. Early Breast Cancer Trialists' Collaborative Group, "Effects of Radiotherapy and Surgery in Early Breast Cancer," *New England Journal of Medicine*, 333 (1995): 1444.

- "A recent meta-analysis of studies of radiation for breast cancer clearly demonstrated increased risks of dying from the radiation compared to the breast cancer itself—in good part due to the negative effects of radiation on the blood vessels and heart."[49]

- "Of the more than 10 million cancer survivors in this nation, those who underwent extensive radiation to treat or find their disease...face lifetime risks of other cancers as a result."[50]

- "The March 1992 issue of *The New England Journal of Medicine* reported that the risk of recurrence significantly increased among women under 45 who chose adjuvant radiation."[51]

- "[T]he vast majority of studies show that radiation cannot cure cancer, and that it does not usually extend life for people with the disease."[52]

No Strength in These Numbers: Hormone Therapy

Hollie's cancer was estrogen receptor positive (ER+) and progesterone receptor negative (PR-). Generally speaking, this meant that her cancer grew in the presence of estrogen (ER+), and did not react to progesterone (PR-). Hollie's cancer also was HER2/

---

49. John R. Lee, M.D., David Zava, Ph.D. and Virginia Hopkins, *What Your Doctor May Not Tell You About Breast Cancer* (New York: Warner Books, 2002), 54.

50. Devra Davis, *The Secret History of the War on Cancer* (New York: Basic Books, 2007), 414.

51. Susun Weed, *Breast Cancer, Breast Health!* (Woodstock: Ash Tree Publishing, 1996), 198.

52. John Robbins, *Reclaiming Our Health* (Tiburon: HJ Kramer, 1998), 230. See also Walt Bogdanich, "Radiation Offers New Cures, and Ways to Do Harm," *New York Times*, January 23, 2010, http://www.nytimes.com/2010/01/24/health/24radiation.html?em.

neu positive (or HER2+, also known as ErbB-2). This means that the tumor tested positive for a protein that promotes the growth of cancer cells due to a gene mutation. HER2+ breast cancers tend to be more aggressive than other types of breast cancer, and have a poorer prognosis.

Based on these diagnostics, Hollie was told by her oncologists that she needed to take five years of Tamoxifen, a hormone therapy used with ER+ cancers. For starters, the World Health Organization's International Agency for Research on Cancer considers the drug Tamoxifen to be a "probable human carcinogen."[53] In addition, according to a study in the *Journal of the National Cancer Institute*, "ER+/PR- cancers are relatively resistant to tamoxifen therapy."[54] And while this study was published in 2005 (three years after Hollie's diagnosis), the study is based on prior clinical data that already had shown that ER+/PR- breast cancers are less sensitive to tamoxifen, and that tamoxifen is less effective on HER2+ tumors. Studies published in 1990,[55] 1995[56] and 2000,[57] all well before Hollie's diagnosis, confirm the finding that the HER2 pathway interacts with the ER pathway,

---

53. http://www.lightparty.com/Health/ProfitBreastCancer.html.

54. G. Arpino et al., "Estrogen Receptor-Positive, Progesterone Receptor-Negative Breast Cancer: Association With Growth Factor Receptor Expression and Tamoxifen Resistance," *Journal of the National Cancer Institute*, 97 no. 17 (2005): 1254-1261.

55. L.D. Read et al., "Hormonal Modulation of HER-2/neu Proto-Oncogene Messenger Ribonucleic Acid and P185 Protein Expression in Human Breast Cancer Cell Line," *Cancer Research*, 50 no. 13 (1990): 3947-51.

56. R.J. Pietras et al., "HER-2 Tyrosine Kinase Pathway Targets Estrogen Receptor and Promotes Hormone-Dependent Growth in Human Breast Cancer Cell," *Oncogene* 10 (1995): 2435-46.

57. M. De Laurentiis et al., "Meta-Analysis of the Interaction Between HER-2 and the Response to Endocrine Therapy (ET) in Metastatic Breast Cancer (MBC)," *Proc ASCO* 19 Abstract 301 (2000).

rendering them tamoxifen resistant. Even more unsettling is the fact that women treated with tamoxifen that had ER+/PR-/HER2+ tumors had a higher likelihood of recurrence.[58]

In other words, one of the treatment components that was *strongly recommended* by Hollie's oncologists would have *increased* her chance of recurrence. As a further erosion of our confidence in conventional treatments, the NCI journal article was pointed out to us by our traditional medicine practitioners, *not* by the conventional physicians recommending treatments.

Conventional Cancer Treatment Ethics

As the case against the conventional cancer treatments became more and more clear to us, we were left with a natural question in our minds: *Why?* Why would an entire medical specialty be peddling such harmful and ineffective treatments? And this is where our spirits really dropped, even lower than they'd gone after finding out about Hollie's cancer in the first place. This is when we realized that we were in the midst of an intense power struggle, one that had long ago corrupted the practice of conventional cancer care.

An astute philosopher once said, "the inescapable fate of all revolutions, [is] the setting up of new tyrannies."[59] Prior to our declaration of war on cancer in 1971, conventional cancer treatment was itself in a battle for survival. For most of the 20th century, conventional cancer treatment was still considered quackery by

---

58. G. Arpino et al., "Estrogen Receptor–Positive, Progesterone Receptor–Negative Breast Cancer: Association With Growth Factor Receptor Expression and Tamoxifen Resistance," *Journal of the National Cancer Institute* 97 no. 17 (2005):1254-1261.

59. Thomas Szasz, *The Myth of Mental Illness* (New York: Hoeber-Harper, 1961), 203.

most *doctors*, and rightly so. The surgeries were brutally disfiguring, radiation was often *instantly* fatal, and chemotherapy drugs hadn't evolved much from the wartime weapons of mass destruction from which they descended. And then we declared war, and at that moment, a new tyranny was established, with the stamp of political and social legitimacy. Not surprisingly, the money soon flowed, and the rest is history. Political entrenchment, cemented by incalculable amounts of money.

Dr. Glen Warner, a long-time oncologist, said, "We have a multi-billion dollar industry that is killing people, right and left, just for financial gain. Their idea of research is to see whether two doses of this poison is better than three doses of that poison."[60]

This is harsh criticism, for sure. But it's important to note that, increasingly, this kind of critique is coming from *doctors* themselves, like Dr. Warner. And as with our research into treatments, the more we looked at the problems of ethical lapses and scientific bias, the worse the picture got. A full exposé of the industry is beyond the scope of this book, so we'll leave it to the reader to draw conclusions about some of the things we found:

- "The *New York Times* disclosed at the end of May 2007 that physicians who prescribe blood-boosting drugs get hundreds of millions of dollars every year in what are called rebates."[61]

---

60. http://www.sourcewatch.org/index.php?title=War_on_Cancer#_note-3.

61. Devra Davis, *The Secret History of the War on Cancer* (New York: Basic Books, 2007), 286. The rebates are actual monetary payments in exchange for doctors using certain cancer-related drugs on their patients.

- "The fact is oncology is a business, as well as the grounds for trying to keep people from dying of cancer. Sometimes, its business side stands in the way of its larger, more noble goals. Those on the front lines today do not necessarily have the capacity or the incentive to be disinterested observers. In the case of these blood-boosting drugs intended to deal with the anemia so common in cancer patients, controlled supplements with inexpensive iron have been found to be as effective in many cases as more costly patented drugs in staving off anemia. But there is little effort to promote this alternative. In the U.S. today, we use three times more of these drugs than in other nations, and spend about five times more on chemotherapy, although our cancer survival statistics are not appreciably different."[62]

- David Kessler, MD, then commissioner of the Food and Drug Administration is quoted in Barron's magazine as saying, "Everything is tainted. Almost every doctor in academia has something going on the side, and I don't know what it is, I don't have the authority to find out. I don't know what they are getting legally as far as financial return, stock, money, whatever. I certainly don't know what they are getting under the table."[63]

- "Some oncologists may be influenced by their financial involvement with the therapies they evaluate or recommend. Every year, the American Society of Clinical Oncology (ASCO) lists such potential conflicts of interest by the hundreds in a 25-page "Disclosure Index" to their Program/

---

62. Ibid.

63. Ralph W. Moss, Ph.D., *Questioning Chemotherapy* (Brooklyn: Equinox Press, 2000), xviii.

Proceedings. I am not saying this is illegal or immoral. But it is a situation that bears close scrutiny, since financial involvement encourages the over-estimation of these drugs' value and an underestimation of the damage they may cause."[64]

- Publication bias refers to when "positive results on drugs are more readily published than negative ones. This is also called the "file drawer" bias, since negative results are more likely to remain locked up in a scientist's filing cabinet."[65]

- "While people may think of the [American Cancer Society] as a foremost supporter of research, in 2005 it reported spending less than 10 percent of its nearly billion dollar budget on independent scientific studies."[66]

- "From homeopaths to midwives, the history of the AMA is resplendent with a long, illustrious, and unbroken tradition of trying to do away with its competition. In each case, the AMA appears to have been motivated more by the desire to monopolize the medical market than by wanting to help people or protect them from frauds."[67]

- "In the United States there are now more people making a living off cancer than dying from it."[68]

The Media

The mainstream media limits its coverage almost exclusively to

---

64. Ibid.

65. Ibid., p. 63.

66. Devra Davis, *The Secret History of the War on Cancer* (New York: Basic Books, 2007), xv.

67. John Robbins, *Reclaiming Our Health* (Tiburon: HJ Kramer, 1998), 185.

68. Ibid., p. 229.

conventional methods for cancer treatment. And when it does give mention to "alternative" treatments, it is with fear and criticism that is not equally applied to conventional methods. In other words, non-conventional cancer treatments are held to entirely different standards. It's not uncommon to hear journalists openly mock them.

As Ralph Moss explains, "News concerning conventional cancer treatments seems to come in two varieties: good and bad. Good news, meaning that conventional treatments work well, often generates widespread press coverage and enthusiastic statements from health officials. On the other hand, bad news, such as the fact that conventional treatments have generally been oversold, usually comes and goes unseen, attracting no media attention whatsoever. An example of the first kind is the recent announcement that for the first time in 70 years, the absolute number of U.S. cancer deaths had fallen. Andrew C. von Eschenbach, MD, director of the U.S. National Cancer Institute (NCI), called this "momentous news." Similarly, Dr. Michael Thun, head of epidemiological research for the American Cancer Society, said it was "a notable milestone." How big was the celebrated decline? Deaths actually fell by a total of 370, from 557,272 in 2003 to 556,902 in 2004. Expressed as a percentage of the total, it represents a drop of seven hundredths of one percent (0.066 percent)."[69]

Our Case

In our view, conventional cancer treatment was, and remains, an industry in turmoil. The "science" that supports it is a shifting sand of

---

69. http://www.cancerdecisions.com/content/view/332/2/lang,english/.

ever-changing statistics that have very little to do with living *well*. The ethical structure of the industry, and its lecherous pharmaceutical industry cohorts, is questionable at best. And all of this is wrapped in a cozy blanket of media and social bias, one that has been carefully knitted by the industry itself, at great expense.

CHAPTER EIGHT

Hollie Was Just "Lucky"

*"I am convinced that you were born under a lucky star and that
star continues to follow you wherever you go."*

—FRIEND

There's a fairly obvious response, on the part of conventional medicine, to Hollie's treatment choice: Rather than making a smarter, safer choice, she was merely lucky. She would have been fine even if she had done *nothing* following her lumpectomy. And to this we say—Thank you for endorsing our treatment decision! This is the counter-argument that proves the very argument (ours) that it's trying to refute. Saying that Hollie was lucky is merely another way of saying that she didn't need the harmful treatments being recommended so strenuously to her in 2002. It's just another way of saying that those treatment prescriptions were *medical mistakes*, and that there was another, safer, smarter option that our doctors simply missed. Worst of all, it attempts to explain away the unavoidable fact that chemotherapy and radiation are this era's version of the radical mastectomy—harmful treatments that for the vast majority of women with breast cancer are medical mistakes, and for which the scientific evidence of effectiveness is vanishingly small, if it exists at all.

And there's another more serious problem with this argument. Namely, it ignores the wisdom that underlies the botanical and nutritional science of Hollie's traditional medicine treatment protocol. The logic behind Hollie's treatment is simple—change the body's biochemistry to make it inhospitable to cancer. And again, the multi-faceted methodology for doing so—targeted, synergistic (and safe!) natural medicines, together with comprehensive lifestyle changes, all built upon a solid foundation of nutritional science—is the result of 5,000 years of accumulated wisdom from a wide variety of medical disciplines. When comparing this to the toxic one-size-fits-all conventional treatments that are foisted upon us, "Hollie was lucky" takes on a disturbing irony: Lucky to have avoided conventional treatments?

But perhaps the most troubling thing about this attitude is the complete lack of scientific curiosity on the part of conventional cancer doctors that it represents. Imagine, for a moment, that you're a cancer doctor, and that your scientific knowledge and training tell you that if your patients don't listen to your advice, they'll die. And then imagine that one of your patients rejects your treatment advice, and lives well to tell about it. Aren't you going to try to find out what that patient did? Are you going to try to add to your knowledge, correcting things about which you were obviously wrong?

And do you know how many of the conventional doctors who knew our story asked us about what we did? Zero. And what about the clear condescension in the "Hollie was lucky" attitude? Many have written about how women in particular are treated when they have cancer—taught to feel victimized, infantile, etc.[70] Where are the congratulations for a young woman who did such an obviously brave thing, and worked extremely hard at following an intense treatment protocol for years, and made a complete lifestyle change as well? At best, "Hollie was lucky" is poor sportsmanship in the extreme. It's walking off the court without shaking an opponent's hand after losing a game to a better opponent. At worst, it represents the callous arrogance of modern cancer treatment.

What if?

A related argument to the "Hollie was lucky" concern is "What if it comes back?" It's a perfectly valid question, and one that probably haunts every person with cancer. But it no longer bothers Hollie. The logic of our healing approach to cancer becomes *even more important* if Hollie's cancer were to come back. Because of her aggressive natural treatment protocol, her body would be as strong as it could possibly be, and the cancer would be at a distinct disadvantage, unlike the typical recurrences that take place following failed conventional treatments, where the cancer is often more aggressive and even drug-resistant as a result of the treatments themselves.

Case Studies

Success is the best evidence against this "lucky" claim, as well as against the snarky "it's not science" claptrap. There are a great many unconventional cancer therapies that cure a great many people all the time. From well-publicized stories like that of Dr. Lorraine Day, to

---

70. http://www.barbaraehrenreich.com/cancerland.htm.

people who've healed themselves with non-conventional treatments around the world, we discovered countless cases of people who have cured themselves of cancer. While we didn't choose from among those various options, we're nonetheless happy to see people heal cancer safely and smartly. The point is, these cases deserve at least as much attention as conventional treatments, if not more.

What we did find is what we consider to be the most leading-edge cancer treatment system available anywhere. As we noted in previous chapters, our practitioners were immensely more sophisticated and scientific than our conventional doctors. The successes they've achieved put the lie to the notion of luck having anything to do with it. And it's important to note, too, that the people who are having success with traditional medicine in treating cancer are usually operating against tall odds. A majority of people who turn to traditional medicine practitioners like ours have already suffered repeated medical mistakes on the part of their conventional doctors, making the recovery journey that much more arduous.

Yet still they succeed. And it can't be emphasized enough—they succeed due to an understanding of cancer that is deeply scientific, historically informed, and collaboratively complete, having evolved from thousands of years of medical knowledge, and via treatment protocols that are highly individualized based on one's biochemistry, cancer characteristics, and other essential traits. Here we include a selection of CNH case studies (drawn from upwards of 1,000 patients treated by the clinic) of some other, *very* "lucky" people. Indeed, many even "luckier" than Hollie!

This first case study demonstrates an alternative approach for the vast numbers of women being over-treated for pre-cancers (DCIS) or very early stage cancers that would be particularly amenable to treatment via traditional medicine:

Patient: 62 year-old female.

Diagnosis: Nothing ("suspicious" mammogram).

Healing path: Patient's yearly mammogram showed some changes in calcifications in her breast. A biopsy was recommended, and one surgeon wanted to remove part of the breast, and another wanted to do a core needle biopsy. But because there was no tumor or mass, there would be a number of inserts into the breast with the needle. Both of these procedures seemed too invasive in the patient's opinion, so she sought out treatment from CNH. One year after being on a preventive treatment protocol, she had one more mammogram, which revealed no changes. She then switched to thermal imaging to monitor both breasts, and there has been no sign of any changes or abnormalities in the four years since she began her traditional medicine protocol. This is an excellent example of conventional medicine's over-treating of "suspected" DCIS ("pre-cancers" that are often harmless), or even Stage 1 cancers.

These next case studies are typical of the kinds of patient who come to the clinic. Nearly all have advanced cancers, and most have been treated ineffectively by conventional medicine, often for many years. And despite these enormous disadvantages, the successes are many, and amazing:

Patient: 63 year-old male.

Diagnosis: Liver cancer with extensive metastases.

Healing path: Given 3-6 months to live by his medical doctors. CNH put him on an intense herbal and nutritional protocol, coupled with targeted chemotherapy based on chemo-sensitivity testing. Patient has been on protocol for four years, and remains cancer-free.

Patient: 29 year-old female.

Diagnosis: Stage 3 non-Hodgkins lymphoma.

Healing path: She has been on a CNH protocol for six years, recently had a baby, and her blood markers remain normal.

Patient: Male in his 60s.

Diagnosis: Stage 4 cholangiocarcinoma (cancer of the bile ducts) with liver metastases.

Healing path: Originally given 5-6 months to live in June of 2005, he is now cancer-free, living a normal life.

Patient: 56 year-old female.

Diagnosis: Stage 3 breast cancer, metastasis to lungs and brain.

Healing path: Came to CNH after adverse side effects from chemotherapy, has been a patient for 10 years, and continues to live well.

Patient: Woman in her mid-forties.

Diagnosis: Stage 4 breast cancer recurrence, following initial Stage 2 diagnosis.

Healing path: Following unsuccessful conventional treatment, came to CNH in August of 2006 upon learning of her Stage 4 recurrence. She now has no signs of cancer, has normal tumor markers, has a high quality of life and no longer has other prior health problems, including lupus, ovarian cysts, and migraines.

Patient: 44 year-old male.

Diagnosis: Esophageal cancer, with metastases.

Healing path: Patient was "failing" conventional treatment, and was given 3-6 months to live. As a result of the chemotherapy, he developed "hand-foot syndrome"[71] and extensive neuropathy. Since beginning treatment at the clinic in December of 2008, he is currently disease-free and has complete resolution of his neuropathy. *He also just climbed Mt. Kilimanjaro.*

Conventional science assures us that there is no cure for advanced (metastatic) cancer. These folks, however, like so many others, rewrote their own obituaries with happy, healthy endings.

---

71. A chemotherapy-induced swelling and peeling of the hands and feet. http://en.wikipedia.org/wiki/Chemotherapy-induced_acral_erythema.

CHAPTER NINE

Fighting Fire With Fire

"Unfortunately, for most of the common cancers that kill people, chemotherapy is not very good."

—DR. ANDREW WEIL[72]

The strategy of conventional cancer treatment can best be described as "fighting fire with fire." There's only one problem. That phrase comes from fighting forest fires, where what you're burning is *already dead*! This disconnect between conventional treatments and the living, vital nature of the human body couldn't have made *less* sense to us when we first encountered it. As our healing journey unfolded, we first had a gut feeling that this was the case. Then, over time, the more we learned about conventional treatments, the more we confirmed the wisdom of this gut reaction. Cancer treatments are applied to living, breathing bodies, not a bunch of dead brush, and those bodies need to continue to live and breathe *well* for many years to come. And with safer, smarter treatments available, like the ones we discovered, it's even harder to find justification for the scorched-earth approach of conventional treatments. In yet another moment of our planets aligning in very

---

72. *Larry King Live*, 3/5/03, http://transcripts.cnn.com/TRANSCRIPTS/0303/05/lkl.00.html.

interesting ways, on the very next day following our decision to reject conventional treatment, an article appeared in *The Wall Street Journal* heralding exactly the future that we were starting to see, one that will not include the current conventional approach to cancer:

"A growing realization that women are being vastly over-treated with toxic and dangerous drugs is prompting a widespread rethinking among doctors about the use of chemotherapy.

For years chemo has been the standard treatment for anyone with breast cancer—and it still is in most cases. But now that women are identifying the disease sooner and living longer, physicians are starting to notice more long-term repercussions from chemotherapy."[73]

From "prevention" to diagnosis, from treatment to recovery—we found that conventional cancer treatments were lacking any of the 5,000 years of deep wisdom about the vitality of the human body that we ended up finding in the traditional healing approach that restored Hollie to a level of wellness that was much better than before her diagnosis.

Prevention

The problems with conventional medicine's approach to cancer reveal themselves at the very earliest possible stage of dealing with the disease, which of course is preventing it from developing in your body in the first place. Conventional cancer prevention can be summarized as follows: *There is none.*[74] What's worse is that

---

73. Susan M. Love, M.D., "Doctors Rethink the Wisdom of Chemo for Breast-Cancer," *The Wall Street Journal*, October 8, 2002.

74. In fact, a friend of ours in nursing school shared with us that, during the oncology rotation of her schooling, her teacher said exactly this—there is no prevention for cancer in conventional medicine.

conventional doctors routinely confuse detection with prevention. It's entirely common to hear mammograms pushed as a form of prevention, when of course they are nothing of the sort. You don't go to your dentist to get dental x-rays to prevent cavities, and similarly x-raying your breasts does nothing to prevent breast cancer, and in fact facilitates its growth.

For example, National Breast Cancer Awareness Month (NBCAM) is touted as a month to focus on preventing this disease from affecting our loved ones, and to saving the lives of those already affected. Did you know, however, that the principal sponsor of Breast Cancer Awareness Month is the pharmaceutical company that manufactures Tamoxifen, one of the drugs used to treat breast cancer?[75] The influence of pharmaceutical companies in the treatment and "prevention" of cancer today is disturbing and dangerous.

Note that NBCAM focuses primarily on detection, and some on treatment. It never gives serious attention to prevention, and it definitely never mentions the contributing environmental causes of the disease. Could this be because the founder of NBCAM manufactures carcinogenic chemicals as well as breast cancer treatment drugs?[76] "National Breast Cancer Awareness Month was established by Zeneca Group PLC, a bioscience company with 1997 sales of $8.62 billion. Forty-nine percent of Zeneca's 1997 profits came from pesticides and other industrial chemicals, and 49% were from pharmaceutical sales, one-third (about $1.4 billion's worth) of which were cancer treatment drugs. The remaining 2% of Zeneca's profits

---

75. http://www.nbcam.org/about_board_of_sponsors.cfm.
76. http://www.lightparty.com/Health/ProfitBreastCancer.html.

derived from health care services, including the 11 cancer treatment centers Zeneca operates across the U.S. The herbicide acetochlor, considered a probable human carcinogen by the EPA, accounted for around $300 million of Zeneca's 1997 sales. Tamoxifen citrate (Nolvadex™), the most commonly prescribed breast cancer treatment drug on the market, accounted for $500 million."[77]

According to the NBCAM web site, it remains "dedicated to educating and empowering women to take charge of their own breast health by practicing regular self-breast exams to identify any changes, scheduling regular visits and annual mammograms with their healthcare provider, adhering to prescribed treatment, and knowing the facts about recurrence." So let's summarize the message of National Breast Cancer Awareness Month:

- Perform monthly breast exams, get clinical breast exams, as well as annual mammograms to try to find breast cancer.

- Once you get breast cancer, listen to your doctors about treatment and do not question the standard of care.

- Understand your risk of recurrence (i.e. understand that the recommended treatments may in fact increase your likelihood of recurrence).

Do any of these items sound like prevention? If breast cancer is such a killer, and if its incidence has risen considerably over the last half century, shouldn't a month dedicated to awareness be focused on *preventing* the disease? If you look broadly at the activities of most breast cancer support organizations, you'll find massive amounts of money spent on supporting the cancer industry. And at best, you'll

---

77. Ibid.

find major conflicts of interest. At worst, you'll see pharmaceutical companies supporting product companies whose products contribute to the very disease that the pharmaceutical companies "treat" with their drugs. One organization that can help you sort through this information is Breast Cancer Action (BCA), and its project, "Think Before You Pink" (www.thinkbeforeyoupink.org). BCA calls for more transparency and accountability by companies that take part in breast cancer fundraising, and encourages consumers to ask critical questions about pink ribbon promotions.

We live in a toxic soup, and the fact that conventional medical practitioners aren't working feverishly to help people focus on prevention is perhaps the clearest sign yet that the conventional treatment system exists for its own good, and not the patient's. Overall, almost half of all Americans will have cancer of some sort. The *incidence* of cancer has skyrocketed across nearly all cancers, and around much of the world, and is projected to get even worse in the future.[78] If you're concerned about cancer, then our best recommendation is to start learning *now* about how to live a healthier, happier life. This is by far the best protection against cancer.

What we learned through our experience—and it's utterly essential that you understand this if you have cancer—is that medical doctors are simply not trained in the 5,000 years of medical wisdom and practices that promote the wellness of the human body and prevent disease. To state it in the most matter-of-fact way, the vast majority of doctors don't offer any prevention strategies because *they don't know any*. In addition, an enormous apparatus of intervention

---

78. http://www.medscape.com/viewarticle/551998.

has been created to support the conventional cancer treatment model, and this in turn has created powerful and deeply entrenched interests working to maintain the status quo. Author John Robbins eloquently describes the overall situation:

"Because our dominant medical system has focused on intervention instead of prevention, growing numbers of people are beset by a host of physical problems and difficulties. Most adults, and even many children, suffer from allergies, headaches, back pain, lack of energy, stiff joints, digestive and respiratory disorders, and problematic emotional states, including periodic depression and anxiety. Most of us don't often feel all that wonderful, yet consider ourselves "normal" because most of the people we know are equally lacking in vitality. Meanwhile, there are massive industries profiting enormously from our over-reliance on drugs, and from our following unhealthy lifestyles that lead to an ever-increasing demand for their services and products."[79]

"The medical paradigm that currently prevails in our society, and which the AMA stalwartly represents, has become so deeply entrenched that we often do not realize that it is simply one option among many. But there are other forms of medicine that represent different ways of understanding life and of promoting healing, and that, contrary to what the dominant medical establishment would have us believe, have demonstrated outstanding records of success."[80]

"[D]enial of the fact that orthodox Western medicine has few answers to cancer keeps a dysfunctional system in place. It keeps

---

79. John Robbins, *Reclaiming Our Health* (Tiburon: HJ Kramer, 1998), 6.
80. Ibid., p. 227.

the public marching obediently and blindly through treatments that often mutilate without providing benefit. It prevents public support for alternative treatment approaches from building to a sufficient level of intensity to create real change…It allows people to merrily munch on their hot dogs and junk food, naively trusting that when they become ill the medical technocracy will be there to take care of things."[81]

In the area of prevention, there couldn't be a more stark contrast between what we learned from traditional medicine, and the deafening silence on the subject from conventional practitioners. Not only did Hollie change her body's biochemistry to make it inhospitable to cancer, but a cascade of other health improvements washed over her as well.

Detection

Conventional medicine's limited appreciation for the body's vitality continues in the cancer detection methods it uses. Chief among these for breast cancer is the mammogram, which is a quintessential example of what's wrong with modern cancer treatment—they're harmful, and not very effective. Stop for a moment and consider the logic of mammograms. Breast cancer is the result of damaged, carcinogenic tissue in the breast. So in order to monitor breast health, we violently clamp the breasts in what can only be described as a vise, and then shoot them full of radiation, which is *highly* carcinogenic? Mammograms are common because…they're common. They're like a celebrity being famous simply for being famous. This isn't science.

81. Ibid., p. 246.

The prevalence of mammograms should not create a bias against safer and more effective monitoring procedures. As we worked to find a smarter, safer way to deal with Hollie's cancer, including detection and monitoring, these are some of the things we learned about mammography:

- "[M]ammography is one of the most oversold and understudied technologies in medical history."[82]

- "Some doctors claim that the amount of radiation in a mammogram is so small that it's more dangerous to fly coast to coast. Not true. One mammogram is not a large amount of radiation, but it is much more than a plane ride. And a mammographic series consists of *four* mammograms. Furthermore, radiation focused closely and directly on the breast tissues is far more likely to initiate cancer than whole-body radiation (such as at high altitudes)." A jet flight of 6 hours = 5 millirads of radiation, but the smallest possible dose from a screening mammogram done with the best possible equipment = 340 millirads of radiation.[83]

- "Both tissue damage and radiation are known risk factors for breast cancer, so it may even be logical to assume that mammography can *contribute* to breast cancer."[84]

- "[R]adiation is a potent risk factor for breast cancer, its effect is cumulative, and mammography involves forcefully

82. Devra Davis, *The Secret History of the War on Cancer* (New York: Basic Books, 2007), 268.

83. Susun Weed, *Breast Cancer, Breast Health!* (Woodstock: Ash Tree Publishing, 1996), 17-18.

84. John R. Lee, M.D., David Zava, Ph.D. and Virginia Hopkins, *What Your Doctor May Not Tell You About Breast Cancer* (New York: Warner Books, 2002), 9.

squashing the breast and then shooting radiation through it."[85]

• "[M]ammography is less useful in most young women, who tend to have much more dense breast tissue than fat."[86]

• "Routine mammography...does not seem to help premenopausal women. False negatives are twice as likely to occur in premenopausal mammograms because of their denser breast tissue."[87]

• "Today mammography is booming. Digital mammography has replaced conventional as the technology most people think is better, but data to prove that this is the case are not easy to find. What is clear is that a digital mammogram machine costs about five times more to purchase and finds many more things that need to be looked at more thoroughly. What is not clear is whether this will lead to fewer cases of advanced breast cancer."[88]

• "Recent drops in deaths from breast cancer have been chalked up to the decline in the use of hormone replacement therapy as well as the increased accuracy of breast screening programs. No mention has been made of the possible role of the hundred-fold lower levels of cancerous pesticides and some key air and water pollutants found in the breast milk of women that has also occurred at this same time. Nor can

85. Ibid., p. 10.

86. Susan M. Love, M.D., *Dr. Susan Love's Breast Book, Third Edition, Fully Revised* (Cambridge: Perseus Publishing, 2000), 125.

87. Donald R. Yance, *Herbal Medicine, Healing & Cancer* (Chicago: Keats Publishing, 1999), 317.

88. Devra Davis, *The Secret History of the War on Cancer* (New York: Basic Books, 2007), 277.

we know whether this decline in breast cancer deaths has anything to do with a reported decline in the proportion of women undergoing mammograms in the past seven years."[89]

The promotion of mammograms is also very revealing about how far conventional medical science has wandered from a focus on real, live bodies, living in the everyday world. Standards of "safety" have been reduced to extremely narrowly focused rules that exist in a reality vacuum. The Environmental Protection Agency has set limits for human exposure to carcinogens such as benzene, vinyl chloride, radiation, etc. (and the list goes on for tens of thousands of such toxic agents). **But the cumulative effect is *never* taken into consideration when these limits are established**. This isn't science (or at least not the kind that matters to actual patients). "[I]t defies common sense and basic biology to assume that just because a single agent looks all right when tested on its own, we can safely encounter hundreds of such materials all at once."[90]

When conventional doctors aren't mistakenly touting mammograms as a form of prevention, they're usually promoting the idea that they're an effective way to detect cancer early, and thus to improve one's chances of surviving the disease. But the evidence that purports to show that this is true is as weak as any in conventional cancer research, and this applies to breast cancer and other forms of cancer as well. As we noted before, what's really happening here is that more sophisticated imaging technologies are helping to diagnose

---

89. Ibid. See also www.medicalnewstoday.com/medicalnews.php?newsid=70889.
90. Devra Davis, *The Secret History of the War on Cancer* (New York: Basic Books, 2007), 7.

more cancers earlier, thus starting the post-diagnosis "clock" sooner, which creates the false impression that people are living longer. Also, earlier-diagnosed cancers and pre-cancers are indeed easier to deal with, and in fact many pre-cancers (such as DCIS) don't need to be dealt with at all, which further skews cancer statistics.[91]

It's also important to point out that the vast majority of studies have 5-year windows. The 5-year view of cancer has little scientific basis, but rather became a de facto standard because crafting studies with 5-year windows became necessary to obtain funding approval for research. Both conventional and traditional practitioners confirmed for us that the 5-year mark, post-diagnosis, has very little importance, scientifically speaking.

There may also be significant gender-bias when it comes to the over-use of diagnostic technology. For example, recently the ACS revised its guidelines for prostate cancer screening because "there's little proof that early detection saves lives. The tests can lead to over-diagnosis and over-treatment of slow-growing tumors that might not have caused any problems."[92] Over-diagnosis and over-treatment have long been acknowledged for breast cancer, which is diagnosed overwhelmingly in women versus men, and yet no such prudence is shown in changing the standard of care for women, as it was for men (prostate cancer is obviously a male-only cancer). In fact, when some researchers recently suggested that mammograms may not be a good idea for large numbers of women, outrage ensued on the part of the breast cancer establishment, even though the arguments

91. John Robbins, *Reclaiming Our Health* (Tiburon: HJ Kramer, 1998), 240.
92. http://abcnews.go.com/Health/wireStory?id=10002084.

for decreasing the use of mammograms are similar to those for decreasing the use of certain screening methods/tests for men and prostate cancer. And yet, there was no such outrage in the case of the revised prostate screening standards. The latter news was very matter-of-fact.

Barbara Ehrenreich has written a scathing piece on this gender bias, if you're interested.[93]

See both Chapter 10 and Appendix C for more information about the safer breast monitoring that we use for Hollie.

Treatments

By nature, Western medicine never seeks to address the root of a health problem. Instead, it only masks the symptoms. Conventional doctors rarely do anything actually to change the underlying physical make-up that allowed disease to develop in the first place. We're sure everyone has had some experience with this. In fact, most of us use this symptom relief model even with everyday health annoyances. If you have a headache, take an aspirin. If you have indigestion, take an antacid. If you can't sleep, take a sleep aid. If you're tired during the day, have some caffeine. But each one of these symptoms, especially if experienced on a regular basis, points to an imbalance in the body.

In one of her many early appointments with her oncologists, Hollie touched on this very topic. Having just begun her research about cancer, she asked one doctor, "Isn't the liver a key component of the immune system?" He confirmed that it is. So she asked, "Then if I have cancer, doesn't this mean that my liver (and other parts of

93. http://www.barbaraehrenreich.com/cancerland.htm.

my immune system) aren't working properly? In other words, if cancer has slipped past my immune system and been allowed to grow, doesn't it mean that my immune system is malfunctioning?" She continued with, "Shouldn't we be trying to *fix* my immune system?" The oncologist had no answers for these questions. He acknowledged that "they were researching these things" and then referred back to the standard of care for treating her breast cancer.

We wrote at length in previous chapters about how poorly we feel conventional treatments are supported by scientific research (especially considering how harmful they are), and here we want to share more of how we viewed the *logic* of conventional cancer treatments. The science behind cancer treatments is typically presented in the form of statistics and studies. The logic is presented in conversations with medical doctors who are attempting to convince you that their treatments are a sensible way to approach cancer. It's probably not necessary to say by now that we were unconvinced!

We began each visit to a conventional doctor's office with a list of questions. Below are a few examples:

1. Can you please direct us to research studies/papers that *clearly and convincingly* document the benefits of chemotherapy?

2. Do you have the names and phone numbers of long-term survivors who have been treated with Hollie's specific chemotherapy regimen, so that we can talk to them?

3. Do you have any research or contact information for patients who rejected your treatment recommendations?

4. What are your thoughts on chemo-sensitivity testing, whereby samples of Hollie's cancer tissue are analyzed to

determine interaction with chemotherapy agents *before* beginning treatment?

5.   What is the survival rate of people who suffer a recurrence?

6.   If there is a recurrence, what do we do then? What about the research that shows that recurrence *after* chemo can be a much harder disease to treat (such as the cancer might develop an immunity of some sort)?

7.   Do you know what the long-term implications of these treatments will be? After all, one of the drugs in her recommended chemo regimen had only been in use for seven years. And another drug, while it had been in use for 20 years, had demonstrated toxicity, including heart damage and second-line cancers. Hollie is only 27 years old, so what health crises would she face over the next 20 years and beyond?

As our conversations with conventional doctors unfolded, signs of trouble appeared immediately. Some of the physicians became visibly annoyed that we were questioning their recommendations at all. One oncologist actually stopped us in mid-sentence, as we requested a follow-up visit in a week so that we could pursue some additional research, and snapped, "Really, what are you going to possibly learn in the next week?" Apparently, the "hasten to 'help'" approach that has supplanted the "do no harm" rule leads to a sharp impatience on the part of some doctors. Isn't science supposed to be patient and dispassionate? Nevertheless, we kept pushing forward with our desire for answers, and other doctors were very polite, and as helpful as they could be, but their answers were in no way reassuring (or even complete or accurate, in some cases).

We were never given very much specific research about the benefits of conventional treatments (question #1), and that's because clear and convincing evidence supporting these treatments really doesn't exist. Instead we were just told repeatedly that the treatments were the standard of care. They kept repeating that Hollie's chances of survival would be improved if she moved ahead with the recommended conventional treatment, and "don't worry about the side effects, we can 'manage' those." This standard of care thing seemed more and more like a request to "Be quiet—we know what we're talking about." But to us, it was like an enormous veil being pulled over what we were increasingly learning was *not* very good evidence to support such treatments. And anybody with eyes can see that the "don't worry" advice about the numerous and health-destroying side effects is just plain dismissive. We can certainly empathize that it must be hard for truly compassionate doctors to prescribe such treatments, but that doesn't make the "don't worry" advice any less insensitive.

We did get the names of 2 or 3 patients in situations similar to Hollie's (question #2), but all were recent or current patients, and none could provide any real-world information to us about the long-term effectiveness (and harm) of the treatments. It seemed odd that there wasn't better tracking of patients on the part of the doctors treating them.

Ok, so, what about the patients who turn down the treatments being recommended (question #3)? For several decades now there has been a steady level of women who reject conventional breast cancer treatments right away. Surely our doctors would be fascinated by these subjects, and would want to track their progress as an immensely important control group against which to compare their treatment advice? Surely there would be formal studies that investigate this most-important set of control subjects? But what we found here was *exactly nothing*, and this lack of even informal curiosity, about people who do "nothing," or who follow "alternative" healing protocols, was nothing short of arresting to us. It was the first clear sign that conventional cancer treatment had elements of almost cultish behavior. And there would be other signs, too.

One oncologist never returned our phone call informing her of our decision to *delay* chemotherapy, nor reached out to communicate with us ever again, in any way. If you don't even talk to patients who reject conventional treatments, how might you ever learn from them, let alone track them?

The more obvious it became that there was limited information and discussion available about the treatments, the more they started to feel like a one-size-fits-all approach. Questions about chemotherapy sensitivity testing only intensified this hunch on our part (question #4). Chemotherapy sensitivity testing entails matching one's actual cancer cells (taken from a biopsy) with multiple chemotherapy drugs in order to identify which drugs will be *effective*, and which drugs will be *ineffective*. In conventional medical circles, it's considered controversial, but once again this reflects the rigidity of the standard of care, which can be difficult to penetrate for new and interesting ideas. In fact, most oncologists refuse to consider this testing and are closed off to the idea of biochemical individuality, even though this testing has been around for many years and even though there are more than 60 independent peer-reviewed papers confirming its validity.[94] In our view, even in cases where it provides marginally useful information, isn't that information worth having? And what about situations where it provides a clear indication to use or avoid a certain cancer drug? But here, we ran into more herd mentality. It was not a part of the standard of care, and not a single conventional doctor of ours recommended it. By contrast, sensitivity testing is used in *every single case* by our traditional medicine clinic whenever it recommends chemotherapy. For our part, chemo-sensitivity testing was a moot point. It requires a fresh tissue sample, and Hollie had already had her surgery. But the larger point remained—the one-size-fits-all versus individualized-care picture was becoming clearer.

One of the most consistent things we heard from our medical doctors was that there is no cure for cancer once it comes back (question #5). It's certainly true that the chance of conventional medicine working with very serious or recurrent cancer approaches zero very quickly. But, no cure? This is really where they started to lose us. This was *patently false* information. People cure themselves of advanced cancer all the time. Our tiny little traditional medicine clinic has done it nearly a thousand times over several decades (see "Case Studies" in Chapter 8), and the world is loaded with similar success stories. And the response to this information by our doctors? "*That's anecdotal.*" Whoa!!! If you have cancer, and you're sitting across the desk from your doctor, discussing your options, do you care if the possible cures for your cancer are proven in federally

---

94. Donald R. Yance, "Botanical Medicine–Case Series Results Using the ETMS" (Presentation at Institute for Functional Medicine conference, 2010).

funded, double-blind studies? If there's a cure for your cancer, but it's "anecdotal"—code word for successful treatments achieved outside of conventional medicine—are you supposed to reject it because it doesn't have a stamp of approval from the AMA? The narrow-minded arrogance of that attitude quite literally took our breath away. The fact that doctors expect patients to care that a cure has their "official" blessing is the most obvious sign of all as to just how far conventional oncology has wandered from a true healing mission.

Continuing on the topic of recurrence (question #6), our probing on this subject led us to discover what seems pretty clearly to be more aggressive, advanced cancers that are caused by the treatments themselves. When cancer recurs following chemotherapy, this obviously means that the treatments didn't work, but what's worse is that you're suffering from a double-whammy. Not only is the cancer back, but it's usually more aggressive, and has often adapted to be more resistant to further chemotherapy. But your immune system is dramatically weakened, thus decreasing even more the chance that you'll be able to get well again. In our view, this was reason to pause and consider this treatment path even more carefully. However, despite agreement by our doctors about the grim situation that is a post-conventional-treatment cancer recurrence, they nonetheless persisted in their "big guns" approach.

Finally, our physicians mostly stared blankly when we asked about the implications of Hollie's young age (question #7). There were no answers to this line of questioning, because there couldn't be any. The drugs in use change constantly, and thus there is literally zero information about the long-term effects of these harmful treatments, in particular on very young patients like Hollie. As Dr. Susan Love notes, "Yesterday's answer may be passé today."[95] It all felt very outdated to us, indeed. It felt very much like Dr. Weil had suggested—medieval.

Recovery

Recovery from conventional cancer treatments is an ordeal in and of itself. And the offer of yet more drugs to "manage" it all, themselves with significant costs and side effects, struck us as self-serving on top of narrow-minded on the part of conventional medicine. As we've noted, the damage done by these treatments was (and continues to be) routinely and dismissively minimized on the part of the modern cancer treatment business in America. And worsening your cancer, or possibly even causing you to die when you might otherwise have lived, is a possibility that's virtually ignored. The litany of problems we were facing after conventional treatment, including an "angrier," more aggressive cancer, was, in our view, an unacceptable price to pay. And we felt this was especially true given the documented marginal effectiveness of the treatments, and most especially given that we were discovering an approach that was so much safer and more effective.

---

95. Susan M. Love, M.D., *Dr. Susan Love's Breast Book, Third Edition, Fully Revised* (Cambridge: Perseus Publishing, 2000), 395.

CHAPTER TEN

Fighting Fire With... Water

"You don't have cancer due to a lack of chemotherapy drugs in your bloodstream, or because you have too many breasts or other body parts.

—DR. LORRAINE DAY [96]

I n 2002, we discovered a new world. Cancer still existed in this new world, but the approach to it could not have been more different as compared with the world of conventional cancer treatments we'd just left behind. Gone were the dangerous and largely ineffective treatments, the widespread medical mistakes in the form of vast over-treatment, the one-size-fits-all medicine. Just as importantly, gone were the "fight!" and "war!" mindsets, with their "break out the big guns" strategies, narrow understanding of human wellness, and, worst of all with their paralyzing fear. In place of all this was a calm, cool, and collected response to cancer, one that drew upon thousands of years of medical wisdom, and one whose treatments were as uplifting as they were effective. No more "fighting fire with fire" in this world. At most, the approach to cancer amounted to fighting fire with...water. But, really, there was no more fighting at

---

96. Lorraine Day, M.D., "Cancer Doesn't Scare Me Anymore," video, http://www.drday.com/.

all. We declared peace on Hollie's cancer.

The prevailing viewpoint in this new world is nicely summarized by Dr. Julian Whitaker, a conventionally-trained physician who has spent the past three decades broadening his horizons to include the vast wisdom of traditional medicine:

"I look upon cancer in the same way that I look upon heart disease, arthritis, high blood pressure, or even obesity, for that matter, in that by dramatically strengthening the body's immune system through diet, nutritional supplements, and exercise, the body can rid itself of the cancer, just as it does in other degenerative diseases. Consequently, I wouldn't have chemotherapy and radiation because I'm not interested in therapies that cripple the immune system, and, in my opinion, virtually ensure failure for the majority of cancer patients."[97]

Perhaps the most important difference between these two worlds is the central role that the patient plays in the process of establishing and maintaining health. In conventional cancer treatment, the patient takes on a passive, victim role from the very outset, accepting that cancer is just something that "happens," and suffering through the often unnecessary and always debilitating treatments. By contrast, we observed patient empowerment everywhere we looked in the traditional medicine world, including a much more involved role in one's healing (which is indeed *required* in order for traditional medicine to be effective). And it's no accident that this translates into successful healing from cancer, given the number of studies that show that patients who are confidently and proactively involved

---

97. Laurens Maas, *The Hidden Cure* (Tucson: Wheatmark, 2009), 24.

in their treatments have better outcomes. Devra Davis, in her book *The Secret History of the War on Cancer*, sums up nicely the "enough is enough" attitude when it comes to taking control of one's health, which is a hallmark of traditional medicine:

"Do we wait for more certain proof about potential causes of cancer, both natural and man-made, and continue practices that have left one in three women and half of all men confronting this illness in their lifetimes? Do we act to avoid those risks that appear avoidable, while science continues its mission of amassing enough data to arrive at unquestionable conclusions? Do we acquiesce to the demand that we can only look at cancer hazards one at a time, even though life comes at us all at once as the ultimate mixture?"[98]

From prevention to diagnosis, from treatment to "recovery"—we found that traditional medicine offered a safer, smarter, more comprehensive, and more individualized treatment approach, drawing upon several millennia of medical knowledge while at the same time *prudently* leveraging the best of what modern medicine has to offer.

Prevention

Unlike with conventional medicine, where preventive efforts and information are virtually non-existent, in the traditional medicine world prevention is the very foundation of wellness. The healing system presented to us included a comprehensive approach to prevention, one that we supplemented over the years as we learned

---

98. Devra Davis, *The Secret History of the War on Cancer* (New York: Basic Books, 2007), 452.

how to establish a true wellness lifestyle.

Diet is one of the most important areas to address in establishing wellness. The human body is the most sophisticated machine in the universe, and yet we don't fuel it accordingly. In 2002, we had a very typical, thoughtless American diet—heavily processed foods, including regular intake of fast foods, massive amounts of sugar (desserts, candy, sodas, etc.[99]), rancid fats, and virtually zero "vital" fuel for the body. We changed all of that, quite literally in one fell swoop. One day, we emptied our refrigerator, pantry, cupboards, even our spice rack, and started over from scratch. We seemingly ate almond butter and raw honey on flax seed bread three times per day for a while, since that was one of the first vital-foods meals we learned to make, but, over time we uncovered a wealth of information about how to eat foods that are delicious and health-promoting. Today, we only eat organic, whole (unprocessed) foods, but every meal feels like restaurant-quality to us. We can't encourage you strongly enough to embrace nutritional science in fueling the amazing machine that is your body, with each and every mouthful, each and every day. This is quite literally the cornerstone of cancer-free living.

Eliminating exposure to toxins is also an essential step for anyone wanting to maximize cancer prevention efforts in one's life. There's simply no denying that we live in a toxic soup. From household to gardening to personal care products, but also including a barrage of environmental toxins (in the air we breathe, water we drink and clean with, etc.), the average person is exposed to dozens or even hundreds

99. The average American eats roughly 150 pounds of sugar every year! http://www.naturalnews.com/009333.html.

of known cancer-causing (or cancer-promoting) chemicals and other substances every single day. As with eating, each and every product you use should be thoughtfully selected for its healthful qualities, and especially including the personal care products that we apply to our bodies every day.

Once we elevated traditional medicine healers to the status of lead oncologists treating Hollie, it only made sense to us to circle back and seek out similarly trained practitioners for our everyday/ongoing health care needs. While living in Santa Monica, our family physician was the Oriental Medicine Doctor (OMD) who first gave us the clinic's book on cancer treatment. Upon moving to Colorado, we sought out the services of a Naturopathic Doctor (ND) as our primary-care family physician, with a supplemental role played by a classically trained Homeopath. We also regularly see a Rolfing specialist and a holistic chiropractor. For diagnostics, emergency/structural problems, or the judicious use of pharmaceuticals where appropriate, we occasionally pay a visit to a conventional family physician. Having traditional practitioners directing your ongoing health needs is an essential element of a good cancer prevention plan, as you'll get much better advice on dietary and nutritional science, safer health-promoting natural medicines, more/better attention, and a host of other benefits beyond what you'll find in a conventional medical practice. And if you find one who's versed in understanding the numerous precursor conditions for cancer, you can develop a maintenance protocol of natural medicines to prevent cancer from ever developing.

If idleness is the devil's workshop, then that's definitely where cancer is made. Innumerable studies have shown that regular exercise is an essential part of maintaining a robust immune system. If you encounter a cancer practitioner who questions the value of regular exercise as part of any cancer-free living strategy, then you should start your exercising right away by *running in the opposite direction!*

Finally, there is the emotional/spiritual aspect of cancer-free living. Stress is a key ingredient in the toxic lifestyle the average person lives. Aside from the vast literature on the cancer-promoting bio-chemical impacts of stress, and the related inflammatory states it causes in the body (which forms a breeding ground for cancer), there is an equally vast and not yet fully understood area of study demonstrating a connection between mind and body. In 50 years, it's likely that what we now call quantum physics will provide a more detailed understanding of the continuum that exists between mind, body, and spirit. For now, suffice it to say that we could all use some additional serenity of spirit in our lives. We became more deeply spiritual during our journey than we'd ever been in the past, and this has been an important part of Hollie's return to health.

An excellent book came out right in the middle of our research for writing this book, and it provides substantial support for these kinds of prevention strategies, not just for cancer, but for disease in general. It's called *The Blue Zones*, which is the term researchers use to describe places around the globe where people live long, disease-free lives. Not surprisingly, the folks who live in these "blue zones" live lives that are essentially blueprints for the prevention of cancer and other illness. The good news is, you don't have to live in a blue zone in order to achieve those benefits. We've created our own little blue zone where we live in Northern Colorado, and you can too. If you do these things, as we and many others have, you will have gone a long way towards making your body inhospitable to cancer, and you'll be living a richer, healthier life overall, too!

Detection

As we noted in the last chapter, we were discouraged by the harmful invasiveness of conventional medicine beginning with the very earliest form of intervention, which is detecting cancer in the first place. We rejected mammography right away due to the exposure to harmful, carcinogenic radiation it entails. Hollie's first and last mammogram was shortly after her diagnosis, in August of 2002. But we didn't want to eschew all modern imaging technology as we watched Hollie very closely in the years after her cancer diagnosis. At first, we turned to breast MRIs, which are a highly advanced form of imaging. These weren't at all common for breast cancer monitoring at the time, but through persistence we eventually got so far as to convince our insurance company to reimburse these tests. MRIs do produce non-ionizing radiation[100] and they require a synthetic contrast agent to aid in the creation of the images. They are also expensive. "[MRI] uses a powerful magnetic field, radio frequency pulses and a computer to produce detailed pictures of organs, soft

---

100. It's important to note that MRI radiation, unlike mammograms and other forms of x-ray, does not produce the harmful form of ionizing (or "hot") radiation that can destroy cells, cancerous and healthy alike.

tissues, bone and virtually all other internal body structures."[101] As such, MRIs do not have the risks associated with mammograms. In addition, MRIs are more accurate in monitoring denser breast tissue, commonly found in premenopausal women. "[MRI is] gaining acceptance as a technique that can identify breast cancer."[102]

We found breast MRI to be an acceptable temporary solution, but we began to search for a truly non-invasive, safe method. And that's when we discovered thermal imaging, which is what we now use today as the sole method of imaging our bodies[103] to provide another "data point" for maintaining a disease-free life.

Thermal breast imaging (sometimes called thermography) looks for signs of a developing blood supply, which all tumors require in order to form and grow.[104] "The use of Digital Infrared Imaging (DII) is based on the principle that metabolic activity and vascular circulation in both pre-cancerous tissue and the area surrounding a developing breast cancer is almost always higher than in normal breast tissue. In an ever-increasing need for nutrients, cancerous tumors increase circulation to their cells by holding open existing blood vessels, opening dormant vessels, and creating new ones. This process frequently results in an increase in regional surface temperatures of the breast. DII uses ultra-sensitive medical infrared

---

101. http://www.radiologyinfo.org/content/mr_of_the_body.htm.

102. Susan M. Love, M.D., *Dr. Susan Love's Breast Book, Third Edition, Fully Revised* (Cambridge: Perseus Publishing, 2000), 139.

103. Patrick gets them too, along with his mother, his sister, Hollie's mother and father, and numerous other people we know, both male and female.

104. It's important to note that thermal imaging is useful for detecting a wide range of health problems, from head to foot.

cameras and sophisticated computers to detect, analyze, and produce high-resolution images of these temperature variations. Because of DII's extreme sensitivity, these temperature variations may be among the earliest signs of breast cancer and/or a pre-cancerous state of the breast."[105]

The goal of mammography, ultrasound, and MRI is to find a physical tumor. On the other hand, thermal imaging searches for heat that is produced by increased blood vessel circulation and metabolic changes associated with tumor growth. "Research suggests that when active cancer cells occupy a space as small as 1/5 of 1mm, or about the size of the tip of a ball point pen, they begin to develop their own blood supply."[106] By detecting such small changes in the blood vessels of the breasts, one can pick up pre-cancerous states, thereby allowing the patient to take proactive measures to improve her breast health and reverse any pre-cancerous conditions.

Thermal imaging is completely non-invasive (and affordable), and thus met our extremely high wellness standards in our post-cancer lives. It's an excellent form of detection, and can give you insights into illnesses developing in your body years before they become serious, and thus there are substantial preventive benefits as well.

See Appendix C for more information about thermal imaging.

Breast ultrasound (also known as sonography) is another safe, non-invasive detection method. It "involves exposing part of the

---

105. www.breastthermography.com.

106. Tirza Derflinger et al., *Better Breast Health For Life* (Louisville: Breast Health Education Group, 2005), 58.

body to high-frequency sound waves to produce pictures of the inside of the body."[107] Ultrasound has been in use for at least 50 years, is a common diagnostic tool, and is relatively inexpensive.[108] Images can reveal structure as well as blood flowing through blood vessels. One of its downsides is a fairly high rate of false positives. Also, the quality of the images depends entirely on the technician, and on his/her ability to perceive an abnormality while performing the procedure.[109] But ultrasound is a safe test, especially for those people who are seeking a second monitoring tool to be used in conjunction with thermal imaging. Ultrasound is especially helpful in finding recently activated pre-cancers that have not yet developed a blood supply discernible by thermal imaging.

Treatment

Without question, the biggest difference in the two worlds we were straddling in 2002 is in the area of actually treating cancer once it manifests in your body. As we've described in detail throughout this book, we began our journey with an intense dissatisfaction with the logic and methods of conventional treatments. The human immune system is an astoundingly sophisticated disease prevention and healing machine. It's essential to preventing cancer in the first place, and curing it once it arrives. Yet conventional treatments are violently destructive of immune function. "Orthodox medicine rarely focuses on the immune system as a means of preventing or curing cancer. In fact, orthodox medicine urges women to detect and treat

---

107. http://www.radiologyinfo.org/en/info.cfm?pg=breastus.
108. http://en.wikipedia.org/wiki/Ultrasound.
109. http://www.radiologyinfo.org/en/info.cfm?pg=breastus.

cancer with techniques known to suppress the immune system."[110]

Today, we have a pretty thorough understanding that the immune system is not one organ, but instead a complicated interconnected network of organs, hormones, and communication signals, and thus there is no one easy fix, no one easy drug to administer via IV, no one pill to pop in your mouth every day. In short, traditional medicine tells us that there is no single cure for cancer. *There are hundreds.* The proper response to cancer is to re-balance this complicated system, allowing it to fight any existing cancer and prevent any new cancer from forming. But despite the mountains of information we encountered that clearly indicted conventional treatments, we still hadn't fully realized how unsophisticated conventional cancer medicine was until we discovered a successful traditional medicine clinic with a comprehensive system for treating cancer in a smarter way. Once we saw the two treatment approaches side by side, it was a *rout.* Once we listened to the symphony of truly integrative and health-promoting oncology, the rest became (and remains) a cacophony to our ears.

The nearly *complete* lack of knowledge by our conventional doctors of any other cancer treatment options was disturbing, to say the least. Not only did they lack knowledge, but they *lacked all desire to acquire knowledge*, instead just robotically citing the standard of care. On the other hand, our traditional health practitioners were able to recite every cancer study that our conventional doctors did, and many more! They used a holistic view of the disease, seeking

110. Susun Weed, *Breast Cancer, Breast Health!* (Woodstock: Ash Tree Publishing, 1996), 79.

to understand the underlying causes of cancer in Hollie's body, the specific biology of her cancer, and the specific internal terrain of *her* body. In fact, our conventional doctors weren't even familiar with many of the tests ordered by our traditional practitioners.

By probing into body system functions, one can identify fundamental imbalances in the body that have led to the development of cancer, and can fix those imbalances, thereby restoring health. We chose not to approach the disease with the standard battle mindset and methodology, such as "kill the cancer" or "win the war." Remember, cancer is not some foreign invader of our bodies. Cancer is comprised of *one's own cells* that have simply gone awry due to an under-performing immune system. But the reasons why an immune system is not working properly vary from person to person, and they must be explored on an individual, case-by-case basis.

The protocol under which Hollie was treated is called the *Eclectic Triphasic Medical System* (ETMS),[111] and it has been developed through more than 20 years of clinical practice on the part of its creator, Donald Yance (or "Donnie," as we call him), at his integrative oncology clinic in Oregon, called The *Centre for Natural Healing* (CNH). Donnie is also the author of the book *Herbal Medicine, Healing & Cancer* (which you'll recall from the "Decision" chapter as the book that formally started us down the path of choosing a cancer treatment based on traditional medicine). As our traditional practitioner at CNH summarizes:

---

111. It should be noted that all holistic practitioners are trained in the triphasic/multiphasic model of healing. The ETMS builds upon this thinking to offer a comprehensive and highly sophisticated healing model.

"In most types of cancer, the tumor will only grow if the internal (bodily) terrain is suitable, and cutting out the tumor is not a cure but a symptomatic treatment. It has been estimated that, by the laws of chance, all people actually produce about 10,000 potentially mutagenic cells every day. Those are normally identified as defective by the immune system and removed. In carcinogenesis, however, some of these "rogue" cells escape detection and go on to form tumors. A strong healthy body in a good nutritional state will be more able to identify mutagenic cells when they arise and to deal with them than can a body whose immune system is weakened by poor diet and other physiological stresses. The nutritional/dietary management of cancer is of supreme importance and great emphasis should be given to it. The general aims are 1) to cleanse the body of any toxins it is harboring that can 'feed' the cancer and 2) to create an environment in the body that is hostile to the tumor development, whilst at the same time enhancing the overall health and well-being of the patient."[112]

When did we know for certain that we'd made the best possible choice? There were two specific moments, actually. One was when we would discuss our treatment protocol with our conventional doctors. From research about the multi-pathway efficacy of botanical medicines, to the litany of tests ordered under the ETMS, and pretty much every traditional medicine topic in between, we began to see blank looks on the faces of those doctors. They simply had no idea what we were talking about. And it's critical to note that this was *not*

---

112. Hollie's herbal oncology treatment recommendations, *Centre for Natural Healing*, 2002.

because it wasn't "science." It was *deeply* scientific in every sense of the word, and in fact that was the second sign that we'd made a better choice. Our traditional medical practitioners were intimately familiar with conventional cancer research; *much* more so, in fact, than our conventional doctors. The most disturbing example was a research study, brought to our attention by CNH, demonstrating that the hormone therapy drug Tamoxifen, which is prescribed to millions of women with cancer, would have dramatically increased Hollie's risk of a recurrence, and thus her risk of dying from metastatic cancer. (See the section entitled "No Strength in These Numbers: Hormone Therapy" in Chapter 7). *The conventional oncologists weren't even reading their own research closely.* For us, this was the final nail in the one-size-fits-all coffin.

Hollie's natural medicine protocol was 100 percent tailored to her body, and her cancer, and was immensely more well-informed and scientific than anything we were offered by any conventional physicians. The protocol was comprised of mostly herbal medicines that had a synergistic action against cancer, supported the immune system, helped provide energy, and balanced hormones. It focused on the bone marrow where the white blood cells are made, the organs of elimination (liver, bowel, and kidneys) and addressed the cancer itself by interfering with its reproductive capability.[113] Examples abound as to the insights the ETMS yielded about the specific characteristics of Hollie's cancer, and how best to treat it. As Donnie wrote,

"There seems to be a relationship between hypothyroidism and breast cancer, and yet the majority of health care providers

---

113. Ibid.

treating breast cancer ignore this. 75% of my clients who have breast cancer also have an under-active thyroid. They have been either clinically diagnosed and medicated; or, are suffering from sub-clinical hypothyroidism. Sub-clinical hypothyroidism for many individuals represents the first signs of thyroid hormone dysfunction. This condition usually involves the hypothalamus/pituitary/thyroid axis, rather than the thyroid gland alone and often goes undiagnosed."[114]

Sure enough, upon testing Hollie's thyroid, she indeed had sub-clinical hypothyroidism. When we asked the endocrinologist in Los Angeles who conducted the test what he thought we should do, he said (and we're not joking here), "Wait until it fails completely, and then come back and we'll put you on thyroid medication for the rest of your life."

Moreover, studies dating back to the 1950s "indicate that low thyroid function (hypothyroidism) predisposes women to breast cancer."[115] According to the ETMS, this was not a pattern to be ignored, but rather the thyroid imbalance was just one imbalance that needed to be eliminated as a stress on Hollie's body and immune system. This in turn would strengthen the immune system, making it better able to heal the body from any existing cancer activity in the body, and prevent cancer from returning.

And the thyroid topic represented just one part of the subtle, interconnected web of details about cancer that the ETMS "sees" (but that is missed entirely by conventional medicine). DHEA is another

---

114. Ibid.

115. John R. Lee, M.D., David Zava, Ph.D. and Virginia Hopkins, *What Your Doctor May Not Tell You About Breast Cancer* (New York: Warner Books, 2002), 65.

hormone linked to breast cancer.

"Numerous clinical studies have shown that premenopausal breast cancer patients have depressed levels of adrenal androgens, specifically DHEA and its sulfated conjugate DHEA sulfate...In premenopausal women, low blood levels of DHEA and DHEAS precede the onset of breast cancer by as much as ten years. Research studies on mice highly susceptible to breast cancer revealed that DHEA effectively prevented the spontaneous development of the disease."[116]

This pattern continued to reveal itself as time went on. To some degree, it makes sense that conventional doctors don't seek to understand cancer in these ways. With the narrow-minded approach of the standard of care, and the limited training in the numerous sciences of human wellness, doctors simply have no use for the results of these tests and inquiries. They wouldn't know what to do with the information once they obtained it.

Where conventional medicine offered harmful, one-size-fits-all treatments with scant scientific support, the ETMS offered a sophisticated, comprehensive, and deeply scientific understanding of cancer, and how best to treat it in a health-promoting manner. Where conventional oncology had an almost obsessive focus on "war" tactics, the ETMS took an approach that combined the prudence of the hippocratic oath with an intricate monitoring program to watch Hollie's progress closely. A brief summary of the "ETMS way" of treating cancer is as follows:

---

116. Ibid., p. 64.

- Casts a *much* broader diagnostic net in order to understand the highly individualized characteristics of one's cancer and the conditions of one's body.

- Measures and tracks a wide array of key markers and growth factors to determine cancer course and therapeutic results.

- Applies a three-part model that analyzes a patient's individual constitution ("Branch I"), the environment in which a patient lives, including environmental exposures, stress, sleep, diet, exercise, and so forth ("Branch II"), and also the specific characteristics of one's cancer ("Branch III").

- Strengthens the patient's constitution and immune system and weakens the cancer, resulting in an increased quality of life and lengthened lifespan.

- Applies botanical and nutritional therapeutics that suppress cancer and increase vital immune system functioning, using primarily (or exclusively in many cases, such as Hollie's) state-of-the-art plant compounds, and new pharmaceutical-grade botanicals, all of which are well-researched to inhibit cancer.

- Focuses on root causes of one's cancer via a close interpretation of a wide variety of symptoms and other indicators.

- Uses non-toxic (or low toxic where absolutely necessary), target-specific cancer suppressing agents, and only selects cytotoxic compounds (synthetic or otherwise) based on a toxicity versus benefit analysis.

Today, a network of ETMS practitioners is being created via multiple levels of formal and rigorous clinical training through The Mederi Foundation. When Dr. Andrew Weil suggests that the future of cancer treatment will look nothing like the medieval methodology in use today, he's indirectly talking about systems like the ETMS. In our view, it represents the future of cancer treatment.

Recovery

This is the most rewarding part of following the healing path of traditional medicine. Recovery begins *immediately*, not after months or years of devastating treatments, and what you're recovering from is cancer itself, *not* from the so-called treatments. In short, there is no recovery because there's nothing to recover *from*. There's just the steady march towards ever-improving health, not just in relation to cancer, but in every aspect of your physical and mental/emotional/ spiritual health.

CHAPTER ELEVEN

She Got Well Again

"Hollie and Patrick's commitment to health is truly inspiring. Their courage to resist the pressures of conventional medicine and choose a path that had many skeptical is something I think about daily. Would I have done the same? Am I that strong?"

—FRIEND

S o the answer to the question that forms the title of this book— You did *what?*—is this: Hollie *got well again*. And she did it by rejecting the best advice of conventional cancer doctors, and living *well* to tell about it. As you may have noticed, we use the term "well" a lot, and there are two very good reasons for this. First and foremost, we want to emphasize that we're *intended* to live well, even when we become ill. The body is immensely capable of being well, even if it falters, if only we'll *allow* it to be. But our modern lifestyle often doesn't allow this, and this is especially true when it comes to treating cancer.

Secondly, we use that word so often because, as much as any desire in writing this book, we want to share with you how well we've lived following Hollie's diagnosis. You can indeed make peace with cancer.

Not that it was easy, mind you. In fact, we can't emphasize enough how much of a thicket we had to work though to get where we are today. Again, when our journey began, we were just a young couple with a new baby, a new mortgage, a husband who worked in software as an independent contractor, a few thousand dollars in spare savings, and not a single, solitary clue about wellness. And we were terrified, not just in the very beginning upon learning of Hollie's diagnosis, but pretty much the entire first year of it all. But taking control of getting well again, and not blindly accepting what turns out to be a very bad case in support of conventional treatments, is the first step towards eliminating that fear entirely. We reached beyond the fear, and found the calming truths of Mother Nature. And you can too. The effort is definitely worth it.

Hollie never once vomited from her cancer treatment. She never lost a single follicle of hair, nor a single white blood cell or platelet. In every way, her experience was the polar opposite of the typical cancer patient. In an especially beautiful and empowering triumph of femininity, her daughters never saw her suffer through what amounts to a brutal punishment of womanhood.

But rather than focus on the things that didn't happen to Hollie, or the things she avoided, we instead want to share the *benefits*, in the true meaning of the word, of her courageous decision to get truly well again.

Insight From a Former Cancer Patient

Before we delve into the benefits of Hollie's decision, we first want to share some insights into what it *feels* like to receive a cancer diagnosis, especially as a young person. It may help others struggling with the initial diagnosis, and it may help those of you who don't know what to say or do with a newly diagnosed family member or friend.

With cancer, the days after your diagnosis are characterized by a numb awareness of what's happening. You get the feeling that people are talking about you like you aren't there anymore. And in a way, you aren't. At that point you've become a statistic. You're part of a machine. The modern cancer treatment machine.

At the time of Hollie's diagnosis, her primary emotion was fear – fear of losing her life, fear of not being able to watch her daughter grow up. The fear was intense and at times crippling. People were constantly reaching out, offering support, and wanting updates on how she was doing. While Hollie wanted to console others and tell them, "Don't worry, I'll be okay," she couldn't do this. Most of the time, she couldn't even speak on the phone. Patrick handled nearly all communications in the weeks following the diagnosis.

Please be clear that all the reaching out by friends and family members actually provided a tremendous support. It was the equivalent to energetic arms holding Hollie up. But much has been written about the need of cancer patients to remove all the "clutter" in their lives in order to focus on living. People with cancer must invest time and energy into relationships that nurture them. They should "put relationships that are toxic on hold."[117] Luckily, Hollie

---

117. Greg Anderson, *Cancer: 50 Essential Things To Do* (New York: Penguin Group, 1999), 140.

had only one or two relationships that had to end. Because one's focus becomes entirely about *living*, everything else becomes superfluous.

Our best piece of advice to those who know someone newly diagnosed with cancer: Offer your support, do it daily if you like. But make it clear that you expect absolutely nothing in return. We had some friends who called every single day to check in on Hollie. They would leave messages offering support, sometimes just reporting on a mundane funny story, but would never ask for a call or email back. They made it known that they were available to help in specific ways, but they never said "so call me back so we can schedule that." Those few that did became an added burden. In general, just be sensitive. Now is not the time for someone dealing with cancer to have to deal with emotional hiccups with friends and/or family members.

Our advice to those newly diagnosed with cancer: Ask for help when you need it! Friends and family typically are desperate to do something, anything, to help.

Hollie's situation also was unique because she was so young, and therefore, most of her friends were young. People in their twenties typically are not thinking about cancer, so it was even more stunning for them to absorb and react to the news. Older generations definitely were more comfortable with the topic because they had more experience with it. We did our best to keep the lines of communication open, because we knew how hard it would have been to be in their shoes.

Mind

When you receive a cancer diagnosis, you know how it feels to have everything you think of as "me" and "today" taken away from you, and how it feels to doubt that there's a tomorrow. The first and most obvious benefit of Hollie's decision to reject conventional treatment was an intense elation. Immediately upon making the choice, her spirit lifted, her energy level increased dramatically, and her days were filled with an empowering sense of self-determination. This was due entirely to the lifting of the emotional and mental weight of the looming conventional treatments, because her natural medicine protocol and dietary changes hadn't even begun yet, and thus hadn't had a chance to affect her in these ways. This was the component of our treatment protocol that addressed the person behind the cancer. Hollie wasn't her cancer any longer. She was back in control of her life, and engaged with deep conviction to getting well again.

When was the last time you heard anyone use the word *elation* to describe the *start* of cancer treatment?

Hollie had an intense, deep-seated intuition from the very beginning telling her that, for her, conventional treatment felt like a mistake from which she wouldn't be able to recover. Much of this likely had to do with the fact that Hollie was now the mother of a newborn child. One of our closest friends pointed us in the direction of some really interesting research about the intuitive powers of new moms. Hollie had an intense desire to live for her newborn child. But more than this, she was cultivating a burgeoning wish to live *well*.

Body

As we've described, Hollie's traditional medicine protocol was intense. More than 70 pills per day, plus teas, tinctures, and smoothies (with numerous additives). The results were immediate, impressive, and lasting. The most important result, of course, was that Hollie remained cancer-free. That result could only be observed over the course of many years, and it has certainly been the most celebrated of all the benefits of her treatment. But it very definitely wasn't the only result. Hollie ceased having migraines, vertigo, hypothyroidism, severe (almost daily) gastrointestinal discomfort, and cysts in various places on her body. Her energy levels increased dramatically, and that's *with a newborn!*

The idea behind our traditional medicine approach was to change the body's chemistry to make it inhospitable to cancer. Hollie achieved that all-important goal, but needless to say the cascade of other improvements in overall wellness were greatly appreciated as well.

Environment

To round out our comprehensive approach to getting and staying well, we also made changes to our overall lifestyle and environment. We tossed out literally every morsel of food in our home, and every ounce of personal care and cleaning products, too. We relearned how to eat, clean, and care for our bodies and home. We also moved to Colorado and completed a green remodel of our dream home, where we still live today.

Spirit

Despite all we've said about the mental and emotional benefits that we gained along the way, the truth of the matter is that deep spiritual change was harder to come by. It took Hollie several years to release fully the relentless fear that cancer represents.

Patrick's realization that this was needed came in the summer of 2007. Having been the "coach" to Hollie in supporting the decision, he had been the pillar of strength and focus throughout the ordeal. But, he also hadn't exhaled in five years, either! Deep within, he felt the weight of a crushing responsibility for Hollie. If she died, it would be *his fault.* The fact of the matter is that this is a common reaction for the partner or caretaker of a loved one. There will always be the thoughts such as, "What if I had guided her down a different path?" However, ultimately it is the patient who makes the final decision, with or without support of those around him or her. But for Patrick, the stress of this existential head coaching job, along with the challenges of leading the software company he had founded at exactly the time of Hollie's diagnosis, were taking their toll.

And so we began in earnest delving deeply into spirituality in 2007, and the results have been even more rewarding than those that flowed from our earlier choices. The fact is that spirituality is not optional when it comes to getting well again. We highly recommend that you devote an intense focus to this most important element of wellness. And there's no need to get caught up in semantics. Prior to Hollie's cancer, we would have described ourselves as "spiritual atheists." Today, we're merely spiritual, in the unique ways that we find moving and inspiring. Call it whatever feels most comfortable to you—Jesus, God, Allah, Source, Universe, Energy, or even quantum space. Just make sure you call upon it.

Michaela Chapin Quinn

In 2006, we celebrated an overwhelmingly powerful completion of the circle, a final sign, in our view, of Hollie's return to health. Our second child, Michaela, was born in May, healthy, and on the floor of our bedroom at home. The only people present were Hollie, Patrick, our midwife, and Hollie's childhood best friend. As Hollie soaked in an herbal bath afterward, we all absorbed the wisdom and capability of Mother Nature that permeated the moment.

In addition to the obvious symbolism for us of having an entirely natural, calm, and confident birth at home, the arrival of Michaela was an important hallmark of Hollie's health overall, since her cancer had initially developed during pregnancy, such that there was a chance that, had her body still been susceptible to cancer, it may well have developed again during a second pregnancy.

Skydiving

After looking back on our experiences since 2002, we tried to imagine a metaphor that adequately describes what it was like to have cancer, and to deal with the fear, complexity, and pressure of making the decision Hollie made. And one that also accurately describes conventional treatments too. In hindsight, those treatments seem surreal to us; surreal that they're the best that medical doctors have to offer in 21st century America. Here is our metaphor:

Imagine you're awoken suddenly and abruptly in the middle of the night, by strangers. You're deeply frightened, yet groggy and disoriented. Somehow, you have a sense that the people who've wrestled you from sleep are well-intentioned, and don't mean you any harm, which gives you a slight bit of comfort. But before you really know what's happening, they whisk you out the door, into the dark of night, and onto a waiting plane, which takes off immediately. The next thing you know, you're in the air, and this is not at all a comfortable trip. It's loud, and dark, and violently tumultuous. There is no illumination in the plane, and no seats. You cling to straps anchored to the fuselage, in the dark. A large door stands open as you fly, allowing in a raging torrent of darkness and noise.

You become vaguely aware that your seemingly well-intentioned helpers are talking about getting you back on solid ground, and appear to know a lot about how to do that. It's hard for you to make sense of anything that's happening at this point, and you're convinced it all must be a nightmare. But the fear is all too real, and all you find yourself thinking about is getting back on solid ground as soon as possible. So you listen, and follow instructions.

They're telling you that you have to jump. You swallow hard, already knowing in your heart that this doesn't seem like the best idea. But your helpers assure you that it's the best known way to get back on your own two feet again, on the ground. Again, in your haze of mortal fear, it's difficult even to process information, let alone to ask questions, and before you realize it, your helpers are fitting you with a parachute made of lead. "Don't worry about that," you're told. "It will open just fine when you jump." "Really?" you wonder? And your helpers proceed to give you a series of statistics that seem to show that jumping out of that plane, with that lead parachute on, is in fact the best idea. The only idea, really.

So you jump. And the ride down is exactly what you feared.

You're going too fast. It's too hard on your body. Your fear builds. As promised, the chute opens, but only partially. And it only slows you down partially. You hit the ground. *Hard.* The fall and landing have taken a lot out of you, but you feel gratitude building inside, knowing that you're still alive, somehow, especially when you look around and notice that many others didn't survive the devastating fall. It's hard to imagine *anyone* could survive that kind of fall. You find yourself filled with a victorious exhilaration. "Hooray!! I made it!" And you look at the crumpled lead parachute lying on the ground, and think, "Good thing I had that!"

The treatments recommended to us in 2002—chemotherapy, radiation, and hormone therapy—seemed like a lead parachute to a skydiver. They just didn't seem to make any sense at all. And they weren't really being offered to us, either. We were told that the best science available dictated that there was nothing to debate. It was a clear-cut, even obvious, decision. We were even told by some doctors, point-blank, that Hollie would die without the treatments. Sure, your helpers will adjust the straps on the lead parachute that is conventional cancer treatment. And perhaps "give you something to help" with the fall and landing. But it's clear—you must jump, with only this lead parachute on, and *quickly*. That sounds pretty convincing, especially when you're not a medical doctor, and especially when you think you're going to die and leave behind a motherless child and a widower husband, which is what Hollie felt pretty much every day in the beginning. But as convincing as it sounded, there was only one problem with the advice given to us by our doctors—it was wrong.

What we learned is that cancer treatment doesn't have to be as damaging as skydiving with a lead parachute. There are lots of different parachutes to strap on if you're unfortunate enough to find yourself on that cancer plane. In fact, you can even take the controls of the plane, and land safely without having to jump at all. It's the most exhilarating feeling of all to guide yourself back to health, whether by jumping and landing safely and softly, or by taking the controls over your cancer, and piloting yourself to healing. It's an emotional and spiritual rush a thousand times more powerful than having survived that fall in the lead parachute, even as incredible an act of endurance as that is for the people who suffer it. One million times more powerful!

We want you to know that you can get back on solid ground—emotionally, mentally, and most importantly, physically—without doing such incredible damage to yourself. And once you've had this softer landing, you can make sure you don't find yourself in that cancer plane again.

A Blessing From Us To You

Our lives today are admittedly a blissful arrangement of health, happiness, and deep-seated serenity. Our journey began where most cancer journeys start—in a thick and dark forest of fear, where you can't see the forest *or* the trees. We slowly but surely cut a healing path to an almost unbearable lightness of being. Our focus now is on creating more and broader paths from illness to wellness, so that others might find a safe passage, as we did. Our first formal effort in this regard has been this book, and we thank you sincerely for reading it.

We leave you with a wish, offered with all the energy we can possibly muster, that you and yours get well again too, whatever it is that ails you, and whatever path back to wellness you choose. And if your intuition is telling you that there's a safer and smarter way back, then we promise you there is. Hollie found it, and you can too.

CHAPTER TWELVE

Appendix A: Treatment Decision

U pon Hollie making her decision to say "No" to conventional
cancer treatment in 2002, we felt a need to try to explain to
our friends and family why and how we'd arrived at that unusual
decision. It was our first brief attempt to answer the question, "You
did *what*?" So we crafted a document explaining the thinking behind
our decision. This book is an extension of these early thoughts of
ours. Below is an exact copy of what we sent out to our friends,
family, and doctors:

October 8, 2002

Treatment Decision

After much research, thought and numerous consultations with
both conventional and CAM (Complementary and Alternative
Medicine) advisors, we have decided to delay conventional treatment
(chemotherapy) indefinitely and instead to implement an aggressive
natural treatment plan. The treatment course we have chosen consists
of a rigorous regimen of herbal medicines and vitamin and nutritional
supplements, all of which have well-documented anti-cancer
synergies, support the immune system (the most important tool in
fighting cancer) and balance hormone levels. The treatment plan also
will include a strict organic, whole foods diet. During treatment, we
will be implementing a very comprehensive monitoring program

utilizing blood test screening and physical exams. If the monitoring reveals anything abnormal (i.e., possible recurrence), then we will revisit the use of chemotherapy. Another standard conventional treatment is radiation, and we are still evaluating its use.

Rationale

Given our analysis of the details of our situation (specific pathology, etc), we believe that an aggressive treatment plan that also *promotes* health is the most reasonable choice at this time. Aggressive conventional treatments may be warranted in the future, and we'll remain open to them where and when appropriate.

We think there is poor justification for the use of chemotherapy in this particular case (i.e., using it as an adjuvant therapy). Some statistics suggest that if Hollie receives no further treatment whatsoever, then there is roughly a 30 percent risk of systemic recurrence (metastasis). Chemotherapy is thought to reduce that risk to roughly 20 percent. In addition, not all cancer responds to chemotherapy, despite its extreme toxicity. Thus, for every 10 women who receive chemotherapy (and who have cancer similar to Hollie's), 7 would have remained healthy without it, 2 would have had a recurrence anyway, and 1 would be spared a recurrence due to the chemotherapy. This means that in 9 out of 10 cases, chemotherapy is either unnecessary or ineffective.

We believe the short term *and* long term (in particular, the long term *unknown*) side effects of chemotherapy are too compelling to ignore at this time. Most importantly, chemotherapy causes a severe depression of the immune system, at a time when immune system restoration is most needed. It also is known to cause heart damage, second-line cancers, possibly more aggressive and/or drug-resistant breast cancer recurrences as well as neurological problems. Also, one of the chemotherapy regimens recommended to us only has been in use for about the past 7 years, and there is little to no research about its long-term health consequences. In sum, we don't believe the effects of chemotherapy justify the marginal benefit of the treatment in this adjuvant setting. (It's very important to note that we are referring to the efficacy of chemotherapy in treating breast cancer. Its efficacy in treating certain other cancers is substantially better.)

In Hollie's particular case, the rationale for using chemotherapy is to destroy any microscopic cancer cells that MAY or MAY NOT be present in the body. However:

1. There is little (if any) compelling understanding of how cancer behaves on a microscopic level, including the significance, if any, of microscopic spread, dormancy periods, etc. We do appreciate the attention paid by conventional advisors to Hollie's specific pathology, but ultimately the recommendation of chemotherapy is a generic treatment plan based on speculation about that particular cancer.

2. Our reading shows that a healthy immune system is equipped to destroy mutated/carcinogenic cells on a daily basis, and that the presence of cancer indicates a failure of the immune system to do so. We intend to do everything possible to restore the immune system to vital functioning.

We are impressed by the attention CAM advisors have paid to the underlying causes of cancer, and to a holistic view of the disease. In general, CAM advisors know a lot more about conventional research than vice versa. CAM advisors have probed much deeper than their conventional counterparts into body system function (such as thyroid) and specific health indicators (such as blood markers/ levels), and into the relevance of these issues to Hollie's development of cancer.

Our research reveals a multitude of factors (both past and present) that have a high likelihood of having contributed to the development of cancer in this case. We wish to correct or remove those conditions with aggressive natural interventions and/or lifestyle changes, coupled with (and followed by) very close screening, rather than moving directly into chemotherapy as a first treatment.

Regarding the question "Why not do chemotherapy AND complementary medicine?" It's important to iterate that we aren't ruling out chemotherapy entirely. What we're saying here is that our considerable research indicates that, given the right circumstances and a viable natural treatment option, one should avoid conventional chemotherapy. The most strident reviews of the efficacy of conventional breast cancer treatment state that there have been no improvements in overall survival rates in the past 50 years.

We believe that Hollie's body needs time to recover fully from childbirth. It is quite likely that the hormonal environment of pregnancy fueled the cancer in this case, so the end of pregnancy may mean the natural slowing or cessation of this causal factor. Also, we don't believe the body is sufficiently recovered from pregnancy to tolerate chemotherapy optimally.

From Hollie...

In summary, I am extremely appreciative of all the time that our conventional and CAM advisors have taken in helping us to make this decision. While not everyone will agree with my decision, each person's knowledge and patience is greatly appreciated.

As an indicator of how serious we're taking our alternative treatment, we've made dramatic lifestyle changes, including converting to an entirely whole-foods, organic diet, replacing cleaning, general household and hygiene products with natural substitutes, implementing exercise and spiritual healing programs and investing in water and air filtration systems (note here that all of this is IN ADDITION to the treatment program itself).

Finally, the ultimate decision to defer to the CAM treatment at this time is one that gives me the most peace. This peace of mind not only is based on diligent research, but it also is based on my own "gut feeling," which I believe to be critical.

CHAPTER THIRTEEN

Appendix B: If You Have Cancer

There has never been a better time to have cancer. Sure, we just spent an entire book describing the rather grim state of conventional cancer treatments, and indeed the case against conventional cancer treatments is strong. But the point of our book is that there is so much more you can do than what's presented to you by medical doctors. What's more, if you take a holistic view of cancer, one that integrates the very best of ancient *and* modern medical wisdom, and one that respects the vital functioning of your body, then your prognosis is so much brighter. You can declare peace with your cancer, and you can get well again, and you can start doing so *right away*.

The following steps represent our suggestions for a process to follow if you currently have cancer. Some of these steps retrace our own path following Hollie's diagnosis, and others we learned over many years of trial and error, and devotion to getting well again, and staying well.

1. Stay calm.

2. Stay calm.

3. Stay calm. Notice a pattern here? It's absolutely essential that you remain calm. The kind of intense fear that cancer elicits causes the very inflammatory stress in your body that fosters

cancer in the first place. If you're wallowing in intense fear, you're quite literally fostering the very thing of which you're afraid. Worse, that fear will lead you to make poor decisions, and those mistakes can quite literally cost you your life. Remember the message that Hollie brings forth from her journey—you can be well again, even if your doctors are saying you can't without their treatments, and even if your cancer is very serious. If you find yourself having moments of trepidation, revisit the "Lucky" chapter to remind yourself of what's possible with integrative, traditional medicine. Even advanced cancers are cured safely and effectively all the time.

4. Seek out expert integrative oncologists. As we've noted, such practitioners may have a wide variety of titles and backgrounds—Oriental Medicine Doctors, Naturopaths, Master Herbalists, Clinical Nutritionists, etc. The titles don't matter. What does matter is that you're under the care of someone whose understanding of cancer integrates as much healing wisdom as possible, and whose treatments are individualized for you, and as safe for your body as possible. Remember, in the future, cancer treatment won't look anything like conventional treatments do today, so if you're being treated by a doctor who's parroting the standard of care (especially with cancers for which it's proven not to work), or balking at traditional medicine because "it's not science," then you're receiving outdated and substandard

care. If you can't find such a healer, then you can contact CNH, the clinic that treated Hollie (www.centrehealing.com, 541.488.3133), to work with them directly, or to ask for an ETMS referral from their growing network of traditional medical practitioners. It's OK to have MDs on your team for diagnostics and other support, but, only if they're truly prepared to support you and your traditional medicine practitioners. Always be aware of the rush to act, and fear-mongering. If you find yourself subject to such pressures by *any* practitioners, fire them immediately and seek better service.

5. *Get* focused. You're going to need a clear, balanced, and calm mind to get well again. You only want to hold one dominant thought in your mind—health! And with this, there will be lots of logistical matters to attend to, such as coordinating appointments with and input from practitioners, making healthful lifestyle changes, and so forth. You need to do all of this with a calm, singular focus on being well. Accordingly, you'll want to eliminate any and all distractions from this goal. In fact, get rid of the word "cancer" from your vocabulary. Don't view yourself as sick. Instead, you're *returning to health*. You're strengthening your body and your immune system, which are by far the most powerful tools at your disposal. Above all else, avoid the "war" mentality, the get it/fight it/battle it/etc. mindset about cancer. These all keep you in a constant state of low-level panic. As we said earlier, it's time to make peace with your cancer, and

the first step in doing so is to rid your mind of its very name, replacing it with a fierce devotion to health.

6.   Start purifying your body *immediately*. Wherever you are in your cancer journey, treatment starts now! Nutritional science is the foundation of any healthful cancer treatment, and your job is to fuel the amazing machine that is your immune system with only the highest-quality nourishments. Eat *only* the purest, vitality-enhancing foods.[118] Every morsel you put into your mouth is a treatment! Similarly, use only safe, natural personal care products, in particular those that you apply to your skin. Avoid exogenous toxins—household cleaning products, gardening products, and so forth. Get some form of exercise, every day. Get lots of fresh air, and connect with nature as often as possible. Sleep in the darkest possible setting you can arrange.

7.   Start purifying your mind immediately (see items 1-3 for a reminder of how essential we believe this to be!). Beyond the more pragmatic focusing of your mind recommended in item #5 above, here we urge you to develop as deeply spiritual a life as you can. *Semantics don't matter.* If you want to call it prayer, then fine. Meditation? Great. Quiet walks along the beach? Same difference, in our view. What's important here is that you slow your mind, and let yourself connect with whatever you consider to be holy and eternal—God, Buddha,

---

118. A favorite cookbook of ours that we discovered along the way is *Nourishing Traditions* by Sally Fallon.

Allah, Mother Nature, The Universe, Love, Abraham, Source Energy, Quantum Space, etc. Whatever you call it, just find it, and let it bring you peace at the deepest possible level. Do something spiritual every single day. Along with this, get rid of toxic relationships. Again, you need a calm, singular focus on wellness, supported by a profound inner peace, and relationships that drag you down run counter to all of that.

8. Get a support system in place. A wise man once said, if you have five *really good* friends, you're lucky. And do you know why he said five? He had only one hand. The point here is that you need to surround yourself with as many truly supportive people as you can, from your boss at work to your Best Friend Forever and Ever, and everyone in between. For all that we've said about positive thinking, we know you're still going to have days when you're afraid. Family members and good friends will help you through these moments, and will support you in all of the wellness endeavors that are part of your healing from cancer, no matter how inconvenient or seemingly unusual. A separate plate of food of only organic, vital foods at a dinner gathering? You need that kind of support. Firing an unhelpful doctor? You need support in doing that if it's necessary. If you don't have friends or family to call upon, contact us (www.youdidwhatbook.com, 970.430.6448), as we're continually adding support resources for those pursuing smarter, safer cancer treatments.

9. *Stay* focused. There are going to be a million distractions from your mission to get well again safely and effectively—social pressures, financial pressures, work pressures, daily stressors, and more. Remember that you only have one thing to hold in your mind: wellness. This is just the final step in the process we've outlined: Stay calm, get expert help, get focused mentally, clear your body, strengthen the soul, ask for help, and, finally, rinse and repeat. In other words, stay the course!

10. Get well again!

CHAPTER FOURTEEN

Appendix C: Thermal Imaging

Thermal imaging is completely non-invasive. It costs approximately $200, and some insurance companies cover the test. "Just as unique as a fingerprint, each patient has a particular infrared map of their breasts. Any modification of this infrared map on serial imaging (images taken over the course of many months or years) may constitute an early sign of an abnormality."[119]

Unfortunately, many physicians either are unaware of this technology, or they describe it as a flawed formed of testing. The latter is due primarily to a single research study done in the 1970s called the Breast Cancer Detection Demonstration Project (BCDDP). In this study, three breast cancer detection methods were studied: mammography, physical exams, and thermal imaging. With regard to the thermal imaging, the BCDDP was seriously flawed in numerous areas. For example, the technicians who performed the scans were completely untrained. In addition, the radiologists that were used in the study had no experience or knowledge in reading infrared images. To make matters worse, proper environmental controls were completely ignored. Thermal imaging is entirely based on temperature, so the temperature of the room during examination is critical to obtaining accurate results. There also were several other

---

119. http://www.breastthermography.com.

major flaws to the study, but we think you get the point that the primary study that physicians typically refer to when it comes to thermal imaging was seriously misleading.

Since the BCDDP study in the 1970s, there have been many large-scale studies performed, as well as advances in technology, making thermal imaging a viable screening tool. The thing we like most about it is that the test has the ability to find subtle changes in the breast, well before a tumor has formed.

After all, most breast cancers have been growing for 8-10 years before they become detectable/palpable. This leaves the patient with the ability to make some proactive lifestyle changes and reverse any early signs of cancer formation.

Despite everything we've written, we still have heard that quality across providers can vary. So when "looking for a service provider near you, consider whether or not the service includes thermobiological, or TH, risk ratings and estrogen stimulation assessment with black and white images."[120] We recommend contacting The Thermogram Center in Colorado for referrals across the U.S.

---

120. Tirza Derflinger et al., *Better Breast Health–For Life* (Louisville: Breast Health Education Group, 2005), 59.

Index

David Kessler, 70, 148

DCIS, 79, 93

Detection, 85, 89-90, 93, 108, 110, 114, 143, 145

Devra Davis, 66, 70-71, 90-92, 105, 148

DHEA, 118, 148

Diet, 43, 104, 106, 115, 119, 133, 137

Digital Infrared Imaging (DII), 110-111, 148

DNA markers, 57, 148

Donald Yance, 40, 114, 148

Dr. Alan Levin, 61, 148

Dr. Andrew Weil, 7, 48, 83, 101, 120, 148

Dr. Glen Warner, 69, 148

Dr. Kenneth Forror, 10, 148

Dr. Lorraine Day, 10, 78, 103, 148

Dr. Susan Love, 9, 28, 34, 36, 51-52, 54, 91, 101, 110, 148

Eclectic Triphasic Medical System (ETMS), 99, 114-120, 141, 148

Environmental Toxins, 106

Estrogen, 36, 67-68, 146

Ethics, 48, 68

Food, 70, 89, 126, 143

HER2+, HER2/neu, ErbB-2, 67-68

Hippocratic Oath, 7, 27, 33, 118, 148

Hormone therapy, 3, 31, 33, 35-38, 43, 67, 116, 130, 148

Hypothyroidism, 116-117, 126

Immune system, 5, 11, 16, 29, 32, 41, 48, 51, 55, 95, 100, 104, 108, 112-

CPSIA information can be obtained at www.ICGtesting.com
Printed in the USA
LVOW07s1841261014

410578LV00001B/45/P

9 780692 009048